A Mindful Path

Exploring Inner Peace Through Yoga's Ancient Teachings

Prof. MARK FANNING

A Mindful Path

Prof. Mark Fanning

A Mindful Path

Table of Contents

Introduction..8

Chapter 1. The Stress Epidemic: Understanding Modern Mental Health Struggles.....................12

Chapter 2. The Origins of Yoga: An Ancient Science for Body and Mind.................................20

Chapter 3. Breathwork and Meditation: Calming Techniques from the Yoga Tradition...................26

Chapter 4. Mindful Movement: Hatha and Vinyasa Yoga for Mental Balance.......................38

Chapter 5. Yoga Philosophy 101: Key Concepts for Peace of Mind................................42

Chapter 6. Managing Anxiety and Depression Through Yoga...59

Chapter 7. Building Resilience Through Pranayama and Pratyahara..........................78

Chapter 8. Yoga Nidra and Deep Relaxation: Restoring Inner Harmony..85

Chapter 9. Integrating Yoga Wisdom into Modern Mental Healthcare..92

Chapter 10. Creating a Personal Sadhana: Establishing an Enduring Mind-Body Practice..105

Chapter 11. The Psychology of Chakras: Subtle Energy Centers and Mental Wellbeing..............118

Chapter 12. Diet and Lifestyle Upgrades for Mind-Body Health..128

Chapter 13. Continuing Your Journey: Lifelong Learning On and Off the Mat............................153

Prof. Mark Fanning

Introduction

Amid the breakneck pace of modernity, declining mental health indicates growing imbalance in society. Rates of anxiety, depression, addiction, and chronic stress continue rising despite material abundance. However, ancient mind-body practices offer holistic solutions to mend wear and tear of turbulent times if adopted sincerely. This book examines yoga's tools for nurturing lasting wellbeing by calming turbulent minds and nurturing resilience even amid upheaval.

Spanning thirteen chapters, the text outlines yoga's origins as a technology for inner peace developed by mystics and priests in premodern India. Early sections decode key tenets of yoga philosophy for managing mental turbulence. We explore the nature of suffering and methods for cultivating witness consciousness to life's endless fluxes and flows. How yoga views the mind, its tendencies towards distraction, and techniques for emotional regulation also receive attention.

Subsequent sections demonstrate yoga postures, breathing exercises, deep relaxation, and meditation to rebalance nervous system functioning for reduced anxiety and depressive rumination. Theories describe how sustained yoga reshapes brain structures and neurotransmitter levels underpinning mood and outlook. We also examine emerging evidence on yoga's clinical effects from scientific studies.

Prof. Mark Fanning

Later chapters guide readers to construct personalized holistic practices integrating yoga tools including journaling, diet upgrades, energy healing, nature exposure, and lifestyle recalibration around rest, relationships, and purpose. This sustainable regimen termed sadhana nourishes mental hygiene over quick fixes or superficial highs. Discussion emphasizes pragmatically adapting traditional techniques for modern life rather than transplanting esoteric religious ideas out of context.

As the book progresses, further topics explore psychological aspects of yoga philosophy for modern times. Namely the chakra system's mapping of consciousness centers in the body and integrating Western psychology lenses with Eastern wisdom. The text avoids commercial caricatures of ancient concepts by sticking to traditional lineages.

Ultimately finding workable stability in the present era demands upgrading operating systems inherited from outdated epochs. Practices potentiated neuroplastic brains thrive through novelty and challenge underscored by connection and meaning. Yoga synchronizes proven self-care with timeless teachings on the nature of self and reality while skirting dogma.

In total, the book guides readers to view yoga as a scientific framework freely adapted rather than a rigid doctrine. The diverse collection of techniques serve self-healing. Beyond mat spaces and studio classes, yoga offers tools to build lasting resilience amid whatever circumstances we face, the true marker of realized practice. Inner peace stems not from outer conditions but mental skills honed through past adversity.

A Mindful Path

By avoiding commercial caricatures while emphasizing customization around essential pillars of wisdom, community, ethics and self-mastery, the text outlines yoga aimed not just for exercise but for realization of latent potentials hidden within conscious embodiment. Hence no strict adherence to Indian cultural vestiges emerges necessary to unlock benefits. Yoga starts precisely where we stand in the present moment. The integration of modern medicine and neuroscience with proven techniques rooted in somatic experience offers a holistic path to sustained wellbeing of body, mind and spirit - the good life always sought but seldom sustained after initial inspiration fades. Through practical lifestyle integration beyond merely metaphysical pondering or physical postures alone, yoga creates alchemy reconnecting us to ourselves and world at large.

Prof. Mark Fanning

Chapter 1

The Stress Epidemic: Understanding Modern Mental Health Struggles

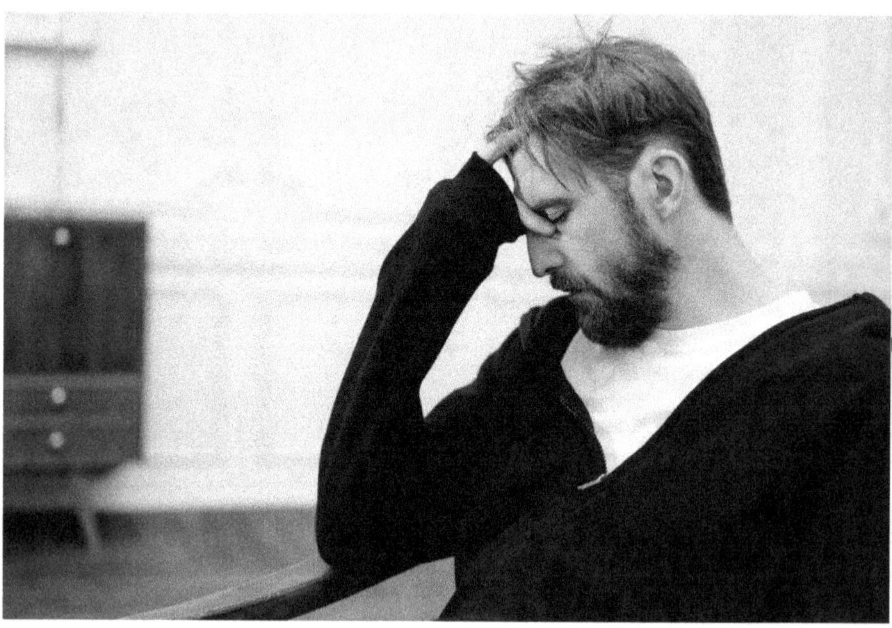

The Calm Before the Storm

It was an ordinary Monday morning when Sara woke to her blaring alarm. As she rubbed the sleep from her eyes and grabbed her phone to check her notifications, she felt a pit in her stomach. Emails had piled up overnight, texts from friends expecting replies, and headlines screaming about political strife and environmental disasters. Her mind started racing about the busy week ahead - work projects to tackle, social commitments to keep, and family responsibilities to manage.

As she dragged herself out of bed and turned on the news, loud voices debated the latest crisis while the weather forecaster declared another heatwave on the way. Her chest felt tight, and her thoughts began to spiral. "How am I going to get it all done? Will I ever find peace amidst all this anxiety and conflict?"

Sara's heart was pounding when she pulled into the office parking lot. She took a few deep breaths to collect herself and plastered a smile as she walked into the office. "Just another manic Monday," she muttered under her breath. Little did she know, a storm brewing would soon be named America's #1 health epidemic - a reality already familiar to millions but just being recognized by health experts and policymakers.

The Startling Statistics

In the 1920s, the leading causes of death were influenza, tuberculosis, and gastrointestinal infections. By the 1950s, chronic diseases like heart disease and cancer dominated. Come the 21st century, psychiatrists made a new declaration: the USA was facing a stress and anxiety epidemic. Over 40 million adults suffer from anxiety disorders, while over 16 million live with depression.

A 2021 Mental Health America survey found that 19 percent of adults had persistent feelings of anxiety and depression, up from 11 percent the prior year. Seventy-six percent of young adults reported mental distress. Shockingly, the US Centers for Disease Control called this a growing "mass trauma event" spurred by COVID-19, political tensions, and climate change worries.

This crisis has spilled into the workplace, too. A Mind Share Partners study revealed that over 50 percent of the workforce suffers from a mental health condition. These individuals struggle to concentrate, make decisions, or interact peacefully with coworkers. Meanwhile, employee assistance providers are flooded by demand.

Clearly, breakneck technological progress has not led to societal improvement. Our fast-paced, hyperconnected digital age comes at a significant cost despite all its conveniences. Facing endless change and uncertainty, many feel disoriented and unable to keep up. Quiet moments for reflection are increasingly rare. With inner peace and mental health taking a backseat, stress now runs rampant.

The Roots of Constant Anxiety

We have underestimated what it takes to maintain well-being in the tumultuous Digital Age. Experts point to three interconnected root causes of this stress epidemic:

The first is Information Overload Syndrome... Understanding Modern Mental Health Struggles":

The Calming Power of Mindfulness

As Sara sat in traffic, she turned on a mindfulness podcast her therapist had recommended. The host's gentle voice soothed her frazzled nerves as he guided a 10-minute breathing exercise. Focusing on the sensation of air passing through her nostrils, Sara felt her tense muscles soften. Her frantic thoughts slowed to a halt. Though the chaos around her continued, she abided in a bubble of calm, peaceful presence. She realized she had a choice - either get swept up in the whirlwind of demands or anchor herself in mindful stillness with disciplined practice.

In Sara's experience, modern life left little room for such pauses. Yet scientists now recognize stillness as crucial medicine for overwhelmed minds. Drawing on ancient meditative traditions, mental health experts endorse mindfulness - nonjudgmental attention to the present moment - to treat anxiety, depression, addiction, trauma, and more. Studies verify its neurological benefits and emotional healing powers. But beyond clinical applications, mindfulness also offers everyday people like Sara relief from persistent stressors through simple, secular techniques requiring no dogma - only an open, curious mind.

Understanding Mindfulness

Emerging from ancient Buddhist psychology, the concept of mindfulness is rooted in the practice of meditation. Meditation trains the mind to increase moment-by-moment, non-reactive awareness of thoughts, emotions, and senses. Daily life tends to draw us elsewhere, caught up in past regrets or future worries while barely noticing the present. By repeatedly guiding attention back to the here and now, meditation builds the muscles of mindful awareness and concentration. Distracting mental chatter gradually settles, allowing a clear-minded presence.

This state of peaceful alertness forms the foundation of mindfulness. Rooted in the stillness of meditation, mindfulness then extends into everyday activity. As we engage with work, relationships, exercise, art, and nature - instead of running on autopilot, we consciously inhibit the moment, mind reconnected to the body in an integrated whole.

A Mindful Path

Cultivating this mindful presence delivers extensive cognitive and emotional benefits validated by thousands of studies. It not only reduces stress and anxiety at the moment but also trains equanimity and resilience over time. Ever-wandering minds become centered. Reactive nervous systems return to baseline. Mental health and life satisfaction improve.

The Neuroscience of Mindfulness

Modern medicine now reveres mindfulness as a powerful therapy. Sophisticated imaging reveals how mindfulness practice structurally changes the brain, creating enduring inner peace.

First, mindfulness strengthens prefrontal cortex activity related to executive functioning - organizing thoughts, regulating emotions, and making decisions. As the observing power of awareness increases, we respond intelligently instead of impulsively reacting. Calm replaces chaotic, scattered thinking.

Second, mindfulness dampens amygdala sensitivity. This neural command center triggers stress and anxiety when perceiving threats. But undisciplined amygdalae often overreact, provoking unnecessary fight-or-flight arousal. Mindfulness soothes these trigger-happy alarm bells.

Third, mindfulness activates the brain's relaxation response by increasing alpha brainwave production. This neural rhythm denotes wakeful calm. Breathing exercises, meditation, yoga, and mindfulness all boost alpha waves. As brain chatter subsides, we enter serene yet clear-headed states, ideal for healing.

Finally, mindfulness shrinks gray matter density in the amygdala while enlarging gray matter in the hippocampus and prefrontal cortex. This benefits learning, planning, perspective-taking, and more - all underpinned by enhanced emotional regulation. The brain rewires itself accordingly as we better handle negative emotions through mindful coping instead of avoidance.

Applied Mindfulness

Beyond restructuring neural connections, mindfulness also develops the skills needed to navigate turbulent times by replacing mindless automaticity with discerning attention. We cultivate curiosity about inner experience, observing how subtle thoughts and emotions provoke significant reactions. Noting tension as it arises, we breathe through it instead of lashing out. Hearing harsh words, we pause instead of retorting. Mindfulness opens space between stimulus and response, empowering wise action. We learn the causes of suffering and how to alleviate them skillfully.

This liberating practice has swept through health care, public education, corporations, the armed forces, and beyond. Mindfulness relieves afflictions from addiction to PTSD. Students concentrate better. Employees communicate effectively, collaborate smoothly, and innovate creatively. Leaders align words with deeds to inspire trust.

Despite changing fortunes, mindfulness helps people greet difficulty with resilience, not rumination. By calmly observing mental reactions instead of getting entangled in them, we experience less emotional turmoil. Equipped with heightened awareness, we understand circumstances clearly to respond helpfully, untroubled by that which we cannot control.

A Mindful Path

Thus mindfulness offers Joe Public the same stress relief once sequestered in Himalayan caves. With simple principles grounded in ancient wisdom yet substantiated by modern science, this convenient, secular technique brings tranquility within reach of all who diligently practice its teachings - something Sara was beginning to realize as she emerged refreshed from her morning meditation despite impending deadlines. Perhaps she could move through the whirlwind not by exerting more effort but by cultivating mindfulness.

Prof. Mark Fanning

Chapter 2

The Origins of Yoga: An Ancient Science for Body and Mind

The Roots of Yoga in Ancient India

Yoga's origins can be traced back over five thousand years ago to the Indus Valley civilization in ancient India. Archaeological evidence shows the people of this advanced culture practiced meditation, ritual bathing, and likely early forms of yoga. Seals depicting figures sitting in meditative postures have been uncovered, giving us a glimpse into yoga's beginnings. Ancient Indian scriptures describe yogic teachings as well, passed down orally long before being recorded in writing.

The Upanishads, composed between 800-500 BCE, introduce vital philosophical concepts of yoga including the idea of the true Self (Atman) vs the ego or individual self. They speak of the mind, senses, and physical body as vessels for the eternal soul. Controlling the mind through concentration, sense withdrawal, and meditation leads one to realize the divine within, according to these sacred texts. The Upanishads planted core ideas about the nature of reality and our innermost essence, which later yoga traditions would draw deeply from.

Prof. Mark Fanning

Between 500-200 BCE, more advanced yoga practices emerged from India's ascetics and forest-dwelling spiritual seekers. Through intense tapas (discipline and austerity), they transform their bodies and minds, developing incredible powers of concentration. Patanjali's Yoga Sutras, written around 400 CE, systemize these practices into an eight-limbed path covering ethical habits, physical postures, breath control, sensory transcendence, and meditation. Together these eight steps aim for samadhi - union with the divine ground of being. This classical raja (royal) yoga provides a framework for psycho-physical transformation that remains influential today.

In the Middle Ages from 500-1500 CE, new styles of yoga arose across India, often centered around a guru teaching specialized techniques. Hatha yoga utilizes precise body postures and breathwork to activate subtle energy channels. The goal is awakening kundalini energy said to reside dormant at the base of the spine. Tantric yoga's transformative rituals and visualization meditations aim at liberating that primal life force as well. Bhakti yoga focuses on loving devotion toward divine incarnations like Krishna and Rama as a path to enlightenment. Jnana yoga finds wisdom through philosophical contemplation and self-inquiry. These schools develop refined yogic technologies while emphasizing different paths suiting students of particular dispositions.

By the 1800s yoga fell out of favor across India due to foreign rule and cultural shifts. But a handful of masters continue to pass down rare lineages. In the early 1900s Indian guru Swami Vivekananda reintroduced yoga to western seekers. His teachings inspire others to spread yoga abroad, sparking a worldwide revival. Yoga arrives as a psychological science for understanding the layers of the mind-body complex while providing holistic healing. Today yoga has blossomed into a full-fledged global phenomenon enriching tens of millions of lives physically, mentally, and spiritually.

A Mindful Path

Modern yoga has its roots in ancient India's remarkable sages, texts, and traditions. Their discoveries about our human potential and how to cultivate greater harmony through self-inquiry and psycho-physical disciplines paved the way for yoga's cosmopolitan flowering we now enjoy. While modern yoga continues evolving, India's rich yoga heritage endures as an inexhaustible fountain of wisdom.

Yoga's Essence as a Holistic Path for Transformation

Yoga's diverse historical threads share a common essence - a vision of human beings as multidimensional creatures with extraordinary potential. Yogic models depict our inner world as far more complex than our surface personalities and social identities. We are vibrant beings composed of interwoven layers of body, breath, mind, intellect, and soul. When these subtle dimensions fall out of alignment, disease and suffering ensue. But the great sages discovered ancient sciences for balancing our many-layered makeup, unleashing deeper aspects of our humanity.

The integrated yoga path works holistically to retune our psycho-physical constitution. By correcting imbalances and removing blockages, yoga allows our innate intelligence, creativity, and joy to shine through. The yogic journey leads from a constricted ego-bound state to an expansive unified consciousness no longer divided against itself. Yoga provides a complete toolkit for self-actualization spanning exercise, breathing, meditation, lifestyle, and more. The many branches of yoga offer diverse skillful means or upayas for unpacking our rich potential according to our unique personality types and proclivities.

Patanjali's eightfold path demonstrates yoga's multifaceted approach working on all parts of our being. The first two limbs - the yamas and niyamas - provide an ethical foundation through vows of non-violence, truthfulness, and other virtues together with self-discipline. Asana or physical postures make up the third limb, enhancing health while reducing anxiety and restlessness. Pranayama breath control directly impacts the state of mind and energy levels by regulating the flow of prana or vital life currents. Pratyahara, the fifth limb, draws awareness inward through conscious sense withdrawal. These stages stabilize the body and mind preparing for the higher limbs.

Dharana, dhyana, and samadhi comprise the inner limbs of meditative absorption. Dharana means concentration - silently witnessing the contents of the mind with non-judgmental attention. In dhyana, unbroken awareness flows centered on one object. As subject/object divisions dissolve, samadhi brings supreme realization of the profoundly interconnected nature of all existence. The eight limbs skillfully develop mind, body, and spirit holistically from the outer sheaths to the innermost core, where yoga's real alchemical magic occurs on the canvas of awareness.

Yoga does not seek to destroy ego, sexuality, or other fundamental human drives that have their own evolutionary utility. Instead, it aims at an enlightened balance where no part of oneself wages war against another. Neurotic compulsions rooted in fear give way to genuine expressions of uniqueness powered by self-love. This permits a natural alignment between inner truth and outer life. Every aspect of the multidimensional system aligns in harmony, manifesting utmost vitality, creativity, and understanding.

Yoga provides a multidimensional evolutionary path engaging all layers of our human system from gross to subtle, outer persona to innermost soul. The integrated approach transforms all parts into a unified expression of wholeness. The philosophy, psychology, and practices contained in the yoga tradition furnish detailed maps of the inner world alongside transformational tools for the journey. While classical yoga concentrates on the transcendence of egoic limitations, contemporary schools also embrace worldly dimensions like relationships, careers, and creative self-actualization.

The fruits of yoga range from improved health and emotional resilience all the way to spiritual liberation or moksha. While classical yoga culminates in a state devoid of all suffering, modern practitioners experience well-being as the embrace of all life's joys and sorrows in a spirit of serenity. Contemporary yoga has evolved into a customized toolbox supporting personalized outcomes. However, knowledge of yoga's origins provides an indispensable context for modified applications. By tapping its ancient wisdom, modern seekers plug into yoga's enduring power as humanity's most time-tested sciences of radically holistic human optimization.

Prof. Mark Fanning

Chapter 3

Breathwork and Meditation: Calming Techniques from the Yoga Tradition

Exploring Breathwork Practices

Yoga reminds us that the breath is our anchor to the present moment. The simple yet profound act of tuning into the natural rhythm of inhalation and exhalation has an instantly calming effect on both mind and body. In the ocean of sensory stimuli and mental chatter we swim in every day, our breath is always there to provide a feeling of grounding whenever we feel tossed about by the waves of modern life.

Most of us pay little attention to this built-in anchor, going about our day on autopilot, unaware of each breath cycle. Yoga teaches us to start tuning into the breath consciously. The more we infuse awareness into every inhalation and exhalation, the more centered and level-headed we become amidst outer chaos or inner turmoil.

Breathwork is an umbrella term for a variety of specialized yoga breathing techniques aimed at inducing relaxation, reducing anxiety, relieving stress, calming anger or irritation, boosting energy, and clearing the mind. Though the methods differ, the underlying premise remains to bring conscious attention to the breath to steer our nervous system away from the fight-or-flight response we habitually get stuck in.

The breath has a direct hotline to the sympathetic nervous system, that luckless part of us that regulates the body's stress reactions. When we perceive threats real or imagined, it instantly signals the release of cortisol and adrenaline through the bloodstream. Heart rate shoots up, muscles tense, blood pressure rises, and breath becomes shorter and shallower as the body prepares to fight or flee. Unfortunately, most of us in the modern rat race live with this threat response turned on all day long, leading to chronic issues like anxiety, insomnia, and inflammation over time.

That's where breathwork comes in as the perfect antidote. Taking just a few conscious deep breaths engages the opposing parasympathetic nervous system instead. Sometimes called the 'rest and digest' function, this calms the body down by lowering cortisol and adrenaline, slowing heartbeat, relaxing muscles, and restoring longer deeper breathing. In other words, it counteracts the fight or flight reaction that poisons both mind and body when we're stressed out. We tap into the body's built-in relaxation response, essentially signaling to ourselves that there is no real threat and we can rest again.

While the experience varies by individual, breathwork typically brings about sensations of warmth spreading through the body, the release of muscular tension, lighter and slower breathing cycles, and a sense of inner quiet permeating one's mental space. This parasympathetic state allows us to think more clearly, make better decisions, access intuition and creativity, strengthen immunity, and gain emotional balance. Pretty nice effects simply from observing the breath!

A Mindful Path

The wonderful thing about breathwork is that it's always available anytime, anywhere. No props, apps, or equipment needed! We carry this portable stress reliever within us at all times. Even taking a minute here and there throughout the day to tune into your breathing can recalibrate your nervous system before emotional reactivity escalates.

Let's explore some of the most time-tested breathwork methods below

Alternate Nostril Breathing—This cooling Pranayama technique reverses fight or flight mode by clearing stuck energy and bringing equilibrium to both sides of the brain and body. Placing the fingers over each nostril, in turn, to guide the breath from side to side has an instantly pacifying quality. Flowing smoothly from left to proper channels and back again improves communication between brain hemispheres while tapping into our whole being. The meditative quality quiets an aggravated mind and flushes out toxic emotions like anger and anxiety. This practice connects us to pure consciousness underlying all mental perturbations. After a session, many report feeling rebalanced, recentered and refreshed.

Ujjayi Breath—Known as the victorious or ocean breath, Ujjayi is another highly effective tranquilizer. Contracting the throat ever so slightly to let the breath flow in and out with a soft ocean wave sound soothes nerves instantaneously. The steady, rhythmic quality and internal resonance induce a relaxation response, great for taming anxiety or anger flare-ups throughout the day. Ujjayi's breath calms the brain, cools hot emotions, and melts away stress, almost like a mini-vacation!

Breath Counts—Counting each inhale and exhale trains the monkey mind to stay focused on the present. Whenever worries over the past or future threaten your peace, return to tallying each breath cycle from 1 to 5 or 1 to 10. The mental effort keeps nagging thoughts at bay while the rhythm of counting in and out further coaxes nervous system balance. Use breath counts anytime during your day as a quick mindfulness reset when you feel your thoughts spiraling.

Breath And Movement—In yoga class you'll experience a seamless dance between breath and body through sequences of postures. Moving through standing, seated, or twisting poses fully immersed in steady conscious breathing unlocks stored tension, leaving you feeling strangely lighter afterward! Intentionally matching breathing to movement helps injury-proof the poses while creating inner stillness as you flow. The breath ultimately leads, and the body follows. Afterward, expect mountain calm and a blanket of inner peace.

Kapalabhati Breath—Want to blast away mental fog or depression? Try a few rounds of the Kapalabhati breathing technique, also known as Breath of Fire or skull-shining breath. Rapid, strong exhalations followed by passive inhalations cleanse the lungs, massage organs, and stoke the inner fire. Expect a burst of invigoration, destroyed stagnation, and awakened clarity! Approach with care though, as too much too soon could leave you drained. When done correctly, Kapalabhati washes through the body and mind like a strong wind scattering clouds to reveal blue sky.

The best part about breathwork is that it becomes second nature to tap into any time with practice. As your awareness muscle strengthens, you'll catch stressful thought patterns faster and course correct through conscious breathing. Imagine being able to head off explosive overreactions, crippling anxiety, or downward mood spirals through something as simple as taking 5 deep breaths! This portable tool alone can profoundly impact relationships, work performance, and overall well-being.

While the above techniques just skim the surface of Pranayama practices, hopefully, you're inspired to explore further. Leading with the breath transforms life's challenges from urgent crises to gentle reminders to realign with presence. Over time conscious breathing crowns us with equanimity, level-headedness, and inner quiet—invaluable allies for thriving in the modern world!

Transitioning from Breathwork to Meditation
As powerful as breathwork is for inducing calm and clarity, the effects tend to come in waves. We ride ascents of tranquil energy and descend back into ordinary consciousness like a sailboat bobbing over the sea. It takes conscious effort to remain aware and focused on the breath rather than getting swept back up by habitual thought loops. Here meditation takes over where conscious breathing leaves off. If breathwork provides temporary glimpses of inner quiet, meditation creates space to anchor oneself there.

Transitioning from Breathwork to Meditation

As powerful as breathwork is for inducing calm and clarity, the effects tend to come in waves. We ride ascents of tranquil energy and descend back into ordinary consciousness like a sailboat bobbing over the sea. It takes conscious effort to remain aware and focused on the breath rather than getting swept back up by habitual thought loops. Here meditation takes over where conscious breathing leaves off. If breathwork provides temporary glimpses of inner quiet, meditation creates space to anchor oneself there.

The Art of Meditation

Prof. Mark Fanning

While yoga and meditation are close cousins, they serve related yet distinct purposes on the inner journey. Both empower self-mastery and resilience when facing modern mental health challenges. However, yoga uses the vehicle of mindful movement, while seated meditation trains stillness and concentration. Athletes flex their physical muscles through training and competition——meditators strengthen their mental focus. Yoga poses engage the senses to create presence through dynamic sequences. Meditation withdraws the senses to cultivate presence free from external input.

So how to define meditation? It's the practice of concentrating attention to heighten awareness, expand consciousness, and align with supreme stillness. The monkey mind learns discipline by repeatedly bringing stray thoughts back to an object of focus like the breath, senses, sound, or phrase. Mental static and disturbances are observed, registered, and released until sense perceptions fade completely. What remains is simple unified awareness resting in its own nature——a field of silent Knowing underlying all sensory experience.

While breathwork delivers temporary glimpses of expanded awareness, dedicated meditation carves deeper grooves to stabilize there. We dip our cups to sample serenity through Pranayama, then learn to swim freely in those tranquil waters through regular practice. Meditation grants full submersion into new states of being far beyond ordinary consciousness. If we dive deep and consistently enough, they become our new normal.

Like exercise for the body, meditation builds 'soul stamina' over time. That is the ability to abide in presence and stillness at will in the face of restlessness, distraction, or dullness. Just as masterful athletes and musicians log endless disciplined hours to perfect their art, meditators also put in the work to master their minds. Without consistent, serious training, the monkey mind stays unruly and constantly gets pulled back into old thought patterns.

While blissed-out meditative states may come and go (and even fade away entirely), the natural fruit lies in how we move through daily life outside practice. When seated with eyes closed, we experience temporary reprieve from input and stimuli, however, chaotic reality always returns post-session! This 'flow state transfer' determines whether meditation makes an actual difference. Ideally, a calm presence cultivated on the cushion permeates all moments off. Calmness and clarity stabilize into our baseline experience as life flows onward.

So, how do we build an enduring meditation practice that transforms our days? Let's break down the key steps:

Establishing Your Own Sadhana

In yoga culture, a sadhana is one's devoted spiritual practice. It provides the container and structure for inner transformation to unfold. Building a personalized daily meditation ritual is the most potent way to reorient the mind away from its usual patterns. Selecting a consistent time and sacred space signals self-care priority while activating the parasympathetic nervous system. We tap our body's natural relaxation response as soon as we sit to meditate.

Begin by contemplating your current lifestyle and responsibilities. When could you consistently dedicate 10-20 minutes to practice daily? Early morning hours before the world awakes tend to provide the highest energy conducive to meditation. However, lunch breaks, before bedtime or even midday, also work. Reflect on your general energy levels during different times of the day. Whenever you feel inspired to devote yourself to sadhana, claim that space!

Next, create a dedicated spot if possible. Choose a quiet room or corner of your home to claim as your temple. Clear out clutter energetically through sagging or prayer if helpful. Some prefer absolute silence during practice, while others enjoy soft, meditative music or nature sounds. Adorning your space symbolically with elements like fresh flowers, spiritual iconography, or candles further sanctifies the energy. This location now becomes your MS (meditation spot) for inner communions.

Prepare as if meeting your most profound love for a silent rendezvous each day. Wash away external energies to receive teachings with a Beginner's Mind. Soak in an aromatherapy bath, self-massage with essential oils, or sip herbal tea to relax body tensions. Release worldly concerns through journaling. Tend bare feet by massaging with coconut oil infused with Arnica and Calendula flowers to soothe nervous system pathways. Slip into comfy clothing without snug waistbands or zippers. Eliminate possible distractions by silencing devices and placing pets comfortably elsewhere.

Set a duration for your practice window, even if short. Use gentle chimes or singing bowls to signify start and finish if helpful. This frames the sacred boundaries of sadhana. Recline comfortably with a spine lengthened. Optional props like meditation cushions, blankets, or blocks allow the body to melt open without struggle. Release jaw, relax hands, and soften gaze either open or closed.

Next comes your meditation method based on personal preference (more details below!) Counting breaths, listening to internal mantras, or sitting in choiceless awareness can all gather stray thoughts inward. Over time, stretch to 20+ minutes to tap deeper states. Track concentration gains and breakthroughs through an old-school meditation log. Note session length, distractions arising, emotions or sensations experienced. Creating your mind training data will help evaluate progress.

Close sadhana with rituals that honor its potency. Offer up intentions manifested into the world through prayer. Bow with hands at heart, sending loving kindness to all. Sprinkle ultra-purified water infused with crystal elixirs to seal new frequencies anchored. Express gratitude for inner access granted each day, no matter how brief. Consider enlivening meditative stillness afterward through dance or song. Finally, enjoy a nourishing meal to integrate expanded energies as they assimilate.

Committing to this daily sacred sequence trains the mind to expect and receive Divine exchange. Whether we label it prayer, manifestation, vision quest, gnostic inquiry, right hemisphere activation, or subconscious rewiring matters not. Meditation provides a portal to ascend beyond ordinary reality. Setting the stage properly says YES to stepping through whenever we need to reconnect within.

Navigating Common Roadblocks

Alas no sadhana journey comes without challenges! Inevitably, we will grapple with procrastination, restlessness, distraction, negative mind loops, and dullness during practice. Some days, showing up at all feels hard-won. Learning to work skillfully with whatever arises transforms each session. Getting disheartened over "failed" sits or berating oneself only reinforces unhelpful mental patterns. Progress unfolds in a spiral fashion rather than linear.

Prof. Mark Fanning

Remember, inspiration waxing and waning is natural even decades into dedicated sadhana. Recognize when your current technique needs modification to pull you through plateaus. Switching it up with alternate focal points can revive excitement like changing fitness regimes ignites enthusiasm. When pure presence without methods feels out of reach, choose structured guidance with props, apps, YouTube visualizations, or pre-recorded meditations. Consider accountability through joining local Sangha circles or mindfulness meet-up groups.

Most importantly, extend compassion to yourself when experiencing setbacks. Our winding path climbing sacred peaks includes slips backward, not just upwards, leaping ahead. Befriending all that arises with patience allows wisdom to dawn organically. Explore thought patterns triggered without self-blame when sessions go awry. Meditation grants a front-row seat to study how the ego operates! Witnessing its sneaky sabotage tactics again and again gradually diminishes its influence.

While a daily formal practice provides immense benefits, casual mini-meditations powerfully reorient the mind, too. Set random alarms on your phone, prompting brief breath counts or inner mantra repetitions throughout busy days. Pause to meditate at stop lights or standing in long grocery store lines. Practice meditation in motion through conscious walking. Leave apps closed and senses minimized for 1-5 minutes between typing emails or text messages. Micro-sessions reset sensory overload from technology and overstimulation.

Through repeatedly returning to sacred practice despite obstacles, inner stillness inevitably blossoms. What once seemed difficult or even impossible effortlessly becomes second nature. We dwell continually in the eye of the storm while life's dramas whirl around the periphery. Attachment and identification with them gradually dissolve until only equanimity shines through each moment. We cherish chaos and confusion equally as portals to realign with eternal peace dwelling beneath it all...

Prof. Mark Fanning

Chapter 4

Mindful Movement: Hatha and Vinyasa Yoga for Mental Balance

In our fast-paced modern lives, many of us struggle to find mental balance. We multitask, switch quickly between activities, and fill any spare moment by checking our phones. This leaves little time for quiet reflection or truly focusing on the present. Practicing mindful movement through hatha and vinyasa yoga can provide that precious time while improving physical health.

Hatha yoga refers to the general category encompassing most yoga styles. It focuses on learning and practicing physical postures while synchronizing breath with movements. Hatha yoga classes tend to have a slower pace with time spent holding poses. This steady effort helps develop awareness both inwardly and outwardly. Tuning into physical sensations, breath, and mental state cultivates concentration skills. Spending time consciously relaxing tense areas counters habitual stress-related patterns of muscle tension. As students learn to release unnecessary effort, the body and mind find greater ease.

Flowing vinyasa yoga coordinates breath with posture sequences, but the pace quickens. Students fluidly move through a series of poses using the power of inhales and exhales. The continual movement patterns challenge the coordination and ignition of proper muscle groups. Athletically inclined students appreciate this style, although teaching should emphasize safe alignment overstraining. The dynamic transitions keep mental focus anchored in the present activity rather than wandering thoughts.

Both Hatha and vinyasa practices guide students to turn their attention inward, sharpen concentration, and inhabit each moment more fully. These are precisely the skills needed to build mental balance amidst outside demands. Yoga's emphasis on self-acceptance and patience, rather than criticism over perceived failures, further bolsters emotional resiliency. Students learn to kindly acknowledge when the mind does wander and then redirect attention to the breath or sensations.

The physicality of mindful movement styles provides a portal for those less comfortable with seated meditation. Exertion followed by rest naturally quiets the mind. Those new to stillness practices often struggle to slow racing thoughts. The gentle pace of beginner hatha courses allows an access point. Incorporating movement with conscious breathing builds the concentration of "muscle" in a supportive environment. Then resting poses reward mental effort while lowering stress hormones. Over time, students grow more adept at settled, focused awareness.

Both Hatha and vinyasa yoga calm the sympathetic fight-or-flight nervous system and stimulate the vital parasympathetic response. These biological shifts signal safety, slowing respiration, heart rate, and metabolism. Regular practice lowers blood pressure and cortisol levels. Anxiety, fatigue, and depression lift with consistent training. Over time, students develop a reservoir of renewal carried into everyday life. The mind and body learn to tap into relaxed yet alert resources in times of stress.

A Mindful Path

The mental balance cultivated by mindful movement schools like hatha and vinyasa yoga cannot remain confined to the mat. Practitioners discover grounded, present-moment awareness as a portable skill. The patient compassion a teacher demonstrates gets transmitted from student to student. These qualities permeate daily interactions with an attitude of dignity and care. Yoga classes build communal bonds from the inside out. The shared vulnerability and support encourage students to extend the same generosity to family, friends, coworkers, and neighbors. In this way, mindful movement ripples out as a force of societal balance and harmony.

Prof. Mark Fanning

Chapter 5

Yoga Philosophy 101: Key Concepts for Peace of Mind

Yoga was originally developed as part of an oral tradition in ancient India where spiritual masters would teach their disciples through first-hand experience, passing wisdom from generation to generation. Only many centuries later were the foundational principles and teachings of yoga eventually codified into written texts. Most key yoga texts were written in Sanskrit, India's ancient language of spiritual scholarship.

Sanskrit words can often encapsulate complex concepts into compact metaphorical teachings that require unpacking to fully comprehend them. Yogic terminology can, therefore, seem dense and esoteric to a modern reader not versed in its cultural context. Yet, at yoga's core, it is an ancient science of the mind meant to cultivate inner peace and self-realization for all.

In this chapter, we will explore key philosophical concepts from Patanjali's Yoga Sutras and unpack how classical yoga teachings reveal a path to understanding our true nature beyond the ego better. Learning yoga's lexicon serves a practical purpose - to provide a roadmap to ease emotional suffering. Let's break down some vital

Prof. Mark Fanning

Sanskrit terminology to comprehend how we can attain clarity and serenity through an inward journey of self-inquiry.

Yoga philosophy rests on the foundational premise that our true essence - pure consciousness or the observing Self - lies hidden underneath a turbulent mind dominated by the ego. The ancient yogis considered this veil of ignorance about our real nature the root cause of existential anguish. To penetrate beneath the uncontrolled thoughts and emotions generated by a restless ego, we must cultivate insight into our soul's innermost workings.

Yoga offers time-tested mental training through a concentrated effort to calm mental fluctuations and ultimately reveal an abiding inner peace unaffected by external situations. Meditation creates clarity as scattering dust motes in a room allows sunlight to stream through a window unimpeded. Core techniques like breathwork, postures, sensory withdrawal, and mantra repetition outlined by the sage Patanjali serve to collect our dissipated energies and reveal the clear light of pure awareness underlying all mental activity.

To comprehend yoga's landscape fully, we must first unpack key Sanskrit terminology central to its philosophy. The Yoga Sutras define five essential principles or Kleshas that encompass the human condition and cause suffering. Let's analyze each Klesha to understand how we can counteract them through self-awareness and progress towards inner freedom or Kaivalya.

Avidya refers to ignorance about the ephemeral nature of worldly phenomena and our true identity beyond physical existence. It sustains Asmita - identification with the individual egoic self or I-ness divorced from universal consciousness. From this distorted sense of self arises Raga - attachment to people/objects that seem to complete us, and Dvesha - aversion towards those that threaten our limited identities. Finally, Abhinivesha denotes an instinctive clinging to mundane existence because we falsely assume death represents complete destruction rather than the soul's liberation.

According to yoga darshana, by clinging to a narrow conception of self, we limit our essential nature and its capacity for unwavering inner peace and pure joy transcending external conditions. Through spiritual practice, we can expand identification with our ego-personality conditioned by life experiences towards connecting with our unconditioned divine essence. Yoga's ultimate goal, or kaivalya pada, involves piercing this veil of ignorance and retracing our awareness back to its unbounded source.

The Yoga Sutras offer a scientifically validated eight-limb or Ashtanga model that encompasses key practices to steadily cultivate a state of meditative absorption or Samadhi. Let's analyze how specific techniques target each self-defeating pattern holding us back from inner freedom.

Yama/Niyama: Ethical personal observances minimize harmful behaviors arising due to greed, anger, etc. Pratyahara: Withdrawing senses from external stimuli reduces clinging attachments/aversions. Asana: Steadies the body and alleviates physiological unease, hampering concentration. Pranayama: Regulates breath/prana, reducing mental agitation. Both promote clarity.
Dharana: Focusing mind unwaveringly inverts habitual outward dissipation of awareness.
Dhyana: Sustained inward absorption expands the limited construct of self/individuality. Samadhi: Complete fusion with cosmic consciousness destroys erroneous identification with ego-personality.

Through dedicated practice, we begin to perceive the ground of Being in which both mind and external phenomena appear and disappear. Yogic awakening entails a fundamental shift in identity whereby we relinquish false notions of selfhood and recognize ourselves in all aspects of creation. We progress through stages where the shadow of ego intermittently reasserts itself before finally dissolving, leaving only soul consciousness untainted by mental conditioning.

Let's analyze two more key terms central to yoga's framework - Vrittis and Kleshas. Examining these indigenous concepts sheds further light on yoga's methodology for uncovering lasting inner peace.

Vritti translates to "fluctuations" or "modifications," denoting the dispersed energy patterns churning within the mind field that continuously shape our mental landscape. Yogic philosophy delineates five chief varieties of vrittis or thought waves the mind constantly generates, absorbing our attention outwardly.

1. Pramana Vrittis correctly decodes any perceived object.
2. Viparyaya Vrittis distorted reality.
3. Vikalpa Vrittis conceives imaginary projections not grounded in truth.
4. Nidra Vrittis operates in dream/sleep states.
5. Smriti Vrittis recollects past impressions stored in the psyche.

Since vrittis originate from sensory experiences processed through mental filters, yogic practices withdraw inward through pratyahara to calm resulting agitations. This enables mastery over our consciousness by marshaling scattered energies inwards through concentration.

A Mindful Path

What precisely induces this unruly flux of vrittis? The five Kleshas comprise innate human afflictions causing avidya or turmoil by limiting soul awareness. Let's closely examine each Klesha to seek underlying drivers.

Avidya describes fundamental ignorance of our true nature as eternal Soul rather than temporary ego-self. This primary misunderstanding causes identification with the limited body-mind organism, which must inevitably age, decay, and die. Not realizing the deathless awareness animating life generates profound fear and insecurity around mortality. Asmita compounds this misperception through attachment to individuality and personality. We become so gripped by the story of "me" that we cannot sense the underlying non-differentiated field of consciousness in which we all share. Lost in separation, avidya fuels endless cravings for pleasant and perpetual stimuli we hope will complete this localized sense of self. We cling desperately to possessions and relationships that seem to promise happiness and stability. Yet when inevitably, these external sources fade away, deep anxiety arises once again. This instinctive but erroneous fear of annihilation after bodily demise further concretes exclusive identity with ephemeral form rather than embracing embodied spirit. Only root insight into our eternal existence beyond mortal frames dissolves this primal ignorance perpetuating profound suffering despite momentary worldly pleasures. By shining light on the timeless awareness of observing all changing phenomena, yoga illuminates that unborn, unchanging essence ever at the core of our being.

The Kleshas mutually reinforce egoic impulses, negating intrinsic wholeness accessible only through non-attached pure perception uncolored by preconceived impressions or memories. For instance, the more we define ourselves based on worldly labels and accumulated past experiences, the more we perpetuate ego-reinforcing habits of craving/aversion.

Overcoming this tetrad of Kleshas is essential before experiential wisdom about our true nature can arise. The eight-fold path of Yoga systematically attenuates these innate human impurities clouding our vision. Regular reflective practice leads to Prati Prasava - the inward introversion of energy dissipated through identification with external phenomena. Gradually, egoic urges subside, no longer reinforced as consciousness slowly divests itself of material entanglements.

Sustained Viveka or non-attached discernment enables direct perception untainted by preconditioning. This concentrated insight consistent with soul wisdom is termed Ritambhara Prajña. Free from self-limiting misapprehensions about reality, consciousness awakens to its inherent attributes of purity, omniscience, and bliss.

The mind can either obscure or reveal its divine source. Another central branch of yoga's philosophical system examines the mechanics of perception, cognition, and resultant suffering. Let's analyze how Yogic psychology explains the genesis of afflictions that distort our self-view and, by extension, our innate capacity for peace.

The main culprit is ignorance about our identity beyond corporeality and habitual attachment/aversion towards external phenomena. Driven by subconscious impurities or samskaras etched into the psyche over lifetimes, the mind projects distorted perceptions colored by past experiences, generating desires for pleasure and security underpinning the illusion maintenance.

The mind superimposes these subliminal activators upon reality, habitually flawing its perceptual register. For instance, seeing a beautiful sunset, mental impressions evoke associated memories, judgments, and emotions that filter direct experience instead of simply witnessing its ephemeral glory in flow with meditative awareness, not clinging to any stimuli.

Such unfiltered absorption of the moment with mirror-like equanimity is soul cognition undistorted by the ego's superficial impulses. Witnessing reality without continually asserting our personality comes effortlessly when mental energy steadies in its source, untainted by latent impressions. This state of unconditioned lucid perception directs attention inward to directly apprehend the formless ground of Being underlying existence - our true nature.

Yogic practices like mantra repetition, visualization and pranayama kindle awareness inward to illuminate the context of exterior flux. Thereby, without escaping our human experience, we become, for the first time, fully capable of navigating it with dispassionate grace, powered by spirit rather than controlled by unconscious complexes.

Over fifteen millennia ago, India's vast heritage of spiritual literature essentially diagnosed humanity's deepest source of suffering - misidentification with our changing exterior self or body-mind phenomena. Yoga's uniquely powerful tools facilitate penetrating this egoic veil to access our soul's radiant stillness, which is always available amidst raging mind-storms.

While exterior transformation occurs in fits and starts through immense effort, interior awakening is our perpetual reality requiring only recollection. This inward journey to soul-rest is reliable when external pillars of identity built on quicksand repeatedly falter. abhisheka trigger: Next time your mind feels besieged by its onslaught of emotions, stresses, and desires, remember you face a choiceless choice - to feed distraction through energetic resistance or recall timeless wisdom already aligned with your true nature's flawless equanimity.

We all possess this inner compass guiding us unerringly to where lasting peace and unwavering meaning await beyond egoic ambition. Yet addictive outward noise often overrides its steadfast signal. What veils soul-sight also illuminates it. By repeatedly gathering fragmented energies dissipated through worldly attachment and directing attention inward, we gradually awaken our consciousness to behold itself fully. ??

This revelatory process for traversing inner territory increasingly concealed by modernity's trance has been meticulously mapped since antiquity. Yoga's treasury of experiential insights refined over thousands of years can reliably steer any sincere seeker toward their sacred destination. Its revelations remain fresh - the joyous homecoming to boundless inner silence, vibrantly conscious of itself alone.??

The wondrous promise of yoga's lifestyle framework is that peace and truth live inside ourselves as our essential nature, not acquired via external conquest. Life's ultimate accomplishment is, therefore, to relaxly dwell in presence, fully awake to reality just as it is. But externalized consciousness habitually grasps experiences to construct reassuring self-images, losing primordial openness that alone reflects the truth. Only discerning interior stillness directly apprehends our limitless whole being always already here and now. This is humanity's spiritual grail sought outside for eons and finally revealed within through yoga's illumined guidance to turn awareness upon itself via mediation's alchemy. Here culminates the soul's epic saga - returning to itself, humility and freedom finally found.

A Mindful Path

Human existence displays a paradoxical dual nature - simultaneously divine and driven by egoic instincts prioritizing self over whole. From this distorted lens, we overlook our unbroken inner completeness. Yoga's practices uncover eternal fullness by dissolving egoic myopia. Gradually, by renouncing limited gratification, wisdom dawns - we already embody the wholeness yearned for through endless becoming.

Yogic teachings possess a timeless resonance in addressing mind-made suffering because they target it at the root - habitual ignorance about our true identity beyond individual selfhood. This forgetfulness generates existential angst and chaotic vrittis together, obstructing our innate stillness and liberating insight. Classical texts prescribe specific methods to illuminate our obscured essence - pure unconditioned awareness beholding but untouched by phenomena. Thereby, yoga facilitates a profound remembering - we already dwell in sacred wholeness with infinite creative potential yet curiously also possess fearful ego-identities perpetually seeking completion despite unconsciously fabricating the separation and anxiety we wish to escape. Untangling this hall of mirrors becomes possible by adopting an earnest path of mindful self-inquiry supported by yoga's illuminating practices and perennial wisdom transmitted from those who traversed its depths to those yearning for life's deepest secrets.

Yoga's eight-limbed framework systematically attenuates conditioned impurities perpetuating a disconnected self-view and resultant anguish. Through ethical conduct, postural stability, controlled breathing, and interiorization of awareness, the mind's habitual outward scattering is progressively gathered, focused, and harmonized. As consciousness introverts through sustained practice penetrating its ground, ego-identification relinquishes along with its attendant sufferings.

Prof. Mark Fanning

When the spotlight of awareness illumines its groundless ground, individual identity founded on mental constructs dissolves. This meditative process engenders a fundamental gestalt shift - from time-bound existence constrained by compulsions seeking ephemeral gratification towards glimpsing our deathless essence invariant across all transformations. Reality unveils its mystical nature as consciousness beholding its manifold expressions while transcending identification with any particular form.

Perennial wisdom transmitted by the yoga tradition affirms that lasting peace and unconditional love abide within as attributes of our true nature. Yet habitually, we search outside ourselves to secure these through acquiring objects or relationships that promise happiness and completeness. By repeatedly turning attention inward through meditative introspection, we learn the art of integration with our essential being, always available though obscured by mental noise.

Thereby inner renunciation of egoic reactions gradually matures into effortless inner freedom as consciousness rests into its unbounded wholeness. Yoga describes this awakened state as Kaivalya - residing in choiceless awareness aligned with our soul's intuitive wisdom. No situation, person, or experience can unsettle abiding stillness once the mirage of a limited self perpetually seeking external security dissolves.

One powerful method for contacting this inner sanctuary is systematically deepening meditative absorption while exploring consciousness beyond conceptual limitations. As attention withdraws from physicality and mentation becomes increasingly subtle, awareness arrives at a threshold between determinate perceptions and their formless source. At this singularity, subject/object duality collapses as attention merges into its unsupported ground.

A Mindful Path

By repeatedly contacting this unified field of pure potentiality underlying mentation, external reality appears progressively dreamlike. The veil of Maya (illusion) becomes perceptible by shining the light of Self-awareness to examine its projections. Thereby, reality's assumed solidity gives way to its inherent insubstantiality. What previously seemed impenetrable, lasting, and important is unveiled as a passing superimposition. This radical shift in perception liberates consciousness by loosening identification with materiality's constraints.

The human mind possesses a divinely bequeathed creative power - what it believes manifests through habitual thoughts, words, and actions crystallizing those seeds into reality. By envisioning higher ideals aligned with soul wisdom through concentrated imagination, past patterns upholding a narrow conception of self gradually unravel to reveal our eternal nature, transcendent yet immanent.

Yoga describes the gateway beyond limited individual existence as Ekagrata Parinama, which translates to "transition towards singular concentration." This culmination stage of meditation ensues when consciousness sheds incessant mental activity to abide as a pure, undistracted being anchored in its formless source.

At earlier phases of meditative training, awareness may contact this ground state transiently before being pulled back into ego-reinforcing vrittis sustaining mundane consciousness. Repeated access inculcates abidance whereby the locus of identity shifts from body-based impulses towards soul-infused perspectives, uplifting our vision.

Prof. Mark Fanning

The initial descent from waking state identity towards accessing subtler realities before complete stillness requires navigating intermediate zones or attenuating sheaths termed Koshas in Sanskrit. These comprise concentric layers of our being spanning from physically dense to increasingly diaphanous. Let's analyze this framework for consciousness to comprehensively understand reality's stratified architecture:

Annamaya Kosha - Grossest sheath intertwined with physical anatomy providing encasement for subtler vehicles holding the soul's energetic imprint animating the body.
Pranamaya Kosha - Underlying sheath of vital life-force diffused as patterns of bioelectromagnetic energies regulating physiological functioning.
Manomaya Kosha - Mental sheath generating thoughts and emotions underpinning ahamkara - egoic identity tying selfhood to mental conditioning.
Vijnanamaya Kosha - Wisdom sheath where higher discernment awakens anchored in soul wisdom rather than intellect/emotions. Enables access to...
Anandamaya Kosha - Bliss sheath represents our essential nature - undifferentiated, unconditioned pure consciousness delighting in its infinitude.

This evocative schema makes experientially palpable the possibility of outgrowing identification with limiting personality constructs toward soul remembrance. By methodically attenuating the sheaths' gravitational pull binding awareness into habitual grooves and ingrained self-definitions, attention eventually rests within its natural state of unconfined radiance.

After that mundane consciousness operating within egoic frameworks no longer overpowers our native state of unified awareness, wisdom, and joy. Rather, moments of clarity and soul-infused perspectives become increasingly frequent. Theophanies once deemed exceptional develop into ordinariness while illusion's hold over consciousness progressively crumbles. Truth-sight takes root.

Spiritual traditions since time immemorial describe rare visionary experiences where suddenly everyday reality's constancy and predictability unexpectedly yield to realizing a miraculous intelligence at its unseen foundation. Yet customarily, such theophanies fade on returning to conventional states, leaving a residual imprint on the psyche. Ancient wisdom lineages sought to encode pathways for rooted awakening - transforming fleeting glimpses into enduring reality.

While revelatory incidents represent a preview of ultimate non-dual awareness transcending subject-object bifurcation, stabilizing this unified vision requires surmounting gravitational tendencies, pulling consciousness back into delusion. By tenaciously cultivating presence and self-reflection to examine conditioned assumptions about identity and the nature of perceived phenomena, egoic veils perpetuating a contracted existence progressively unravel before the steady gaze of meditative insight. Thereby, momentary glimpses blossom into abiding transformation through dedicated perseverance.

But even earnest seekers attempting to foster uninterrupted unity-sight may experience ego backlash due to subconscious resistance towards moving away from once familiar moorings now destabilized by alien vistas of being never imagined. The inner terrain progressively unveils itself to be far more malleable, magical, and mystical than previously conceived by mainstream frameworks. The indestructible sense of individuality, considered our ultimate security, also faces dissolution before the rising tide of universality is apprehended directly rather than conceptually.

Faced with the underside of wonder and terror alike in experiencing reality's uncharted territories, heroic courage is necessitated for consciousness to steadfastly expand beyond its conventional circumference without retreating into sanitized normalcy. Stabilization of unitive insight only blossoms through repeatedly confronting and moving through fear towards the naked embrace of the present mystery in all its raw majesty. No matter how turbulent the intermediate phases are, abiding peace awaits those unwaveringly anchored in truth.

While classical texts cryptically describe meditation's final phases esoterically, the journey culminates in complete unification where consciousness expands to merge into an infinite ocean of bliss from which all existence arises, abides, and finally dissolves. Seemingly disparate phenomena once projected externally, are suddenly realized to appear from within non-local awareness beyond space-time while beholding the cosmic panorama. This implosion of perspective destroys habitual subject-object appearance, revealing a majestic indivisible unicity as the sole reality there is or ever was.

The path leads consciousness, experientially tracing its ascendance through ever more subtle sheaths before finally dissolving even the most diaphanous enclosure to explode into infinity. As layer after layer of identity is shed, the inner terrain changes beyond recognition until nothing conceivable remains to bind awareness even as an invisible presence saves pure subjectivity alone, knowing itself by itself.

Language falters in capturing this ultimate seeing where consciousness somehow beholds the entire external panoply of creation and emerges from within itself while transcendentally grounded in a formless being. Description can only point symbolically. To stabilize this pinnacle, the mystic path offers an enduring realization rather than a temporary intoxicant, which requires giving over limited existence unreservedly through relentless surrender till no residue of ergodicity remains by which to reference relative existence. The soul's destiny is to wake up from all becoming a pure being - its original nature.

While such rarified heights of awakening appear incredibly challenging at our ordinary human stage, where we constantly struggle with baser tendencies, meditation's lower rungs confer enormous benefits in perceptibly alleviating suffering. Regular withdrawal and introspection gradually disentangle attachment from external scenarios as a reflex towards looking within to marshal awareness. By thus learning to regulate attention inwardly, we gain increasing access to our native poise.

Progressively, consciousness relies less on phenomena for security as the focus shifts to connecting with the source, becoming perceptibly more easeful. Gradually, by detachment from mental noise and realizing silence as identity, life unfolds more magically and meaningfully. Daily existence is infused with transcendent glimpses of grace, interconnection, and hidden patterning whereas before we perceived only dead matter awaiting exploitation. Mundanity seen through ego-lenses thus transforms into transparency through which infinity shines.

The key insight meditation bestows is that consciousness creates reality through beliefs held by mass intention. By transforming individual vision rooted in wholeness rather than isolation, each awakened person's presence powerfully elevates collective thought fields towards unity. Thereby, evolutionary transformation becomes seeded through raised frequencies despite external chaos. The choice to turn attention upon itself and dissolve illusion becomes the ultimate responsibility and opportunity during epochs of planetary crisis. Thus, seeking inner stability makes one an emissary of peace and an agent of global redemption more potent than any worldly contribution.

58

Chapter 6

Managing Anxiety and Depression Through Yoga

The Science of Stilling the Mind

While many turn to pharmaccutical solutions for managing mental health challenges like anxiety and depression, the ancient wisdom of yoga offers a more natural way to calm a racing mind and lift a tired spirit. Householders and sages have practiced techniques for steadying the senses and inducing inner tranquillity for thousands of years in India.

Through the synergistic impact of physical postures and breathwork, meditation, and mindfulness, we can rebalance our nervous system, relieve emotional turbulence from the inside out, and seed new mental patterns of ease and optimism. Just as the mind influences the body, so does the body shape the mind. By consciously cultivating this holistic mind-body connection with patience and self-compassion, we discover profound stillness and awakening—even amid the seeming chaos of modern life with all its pressures and stresses.

As we open our hearts with courage through this yogic journey of self-healing, external triggers, and habitual reactions tend to lose power. We reconnect to our wise inner voice as our harshest critic dissolves. By shifting our perspective from "What's wrong with me?"

to a spirit of open-minded inquiry, old wounds lose their sting, anxious what-ifs clear like fog by the warmth of dawn. With dedicated practice, we learn to turn inward and access our vital life force energy. Our breathing settles as our nervous system resets. Over time, a deep calm becomes our new baseline.

There's neuroscience evidence showing why yoga works. Studies indicate it stimulates restorative gamma-aminobutyric acid (GABA) production in the brain, reducing anxiety and depression. Movement, breathing exercises, and meditation techniques promote alpha and theta brain waves, nudging us from hyper-alert sympathetic fight-or-flight dominance into restful, rejuvenating parasympathetic mode. As we cultivate conscious body awareness while quieting our racing thoughts, we tap into the timeless power of presence.

This chapter will explore key yoga tools for managing anxiety and depression, drawing on various techniques that help induce serenity by balancing nervous system activity, stabilizing mood, relieving muscle tension, easing constricted breathing, quieting mental chatter and worry, and increasing our capacity for relaxation. We'll start by using physical postures to calm the body, then explore breathwork before transitioning into seated and walking meditation for calming the mind.

Postures for Soothing Emotional Turmoil

Yoga postures can be very effective for relieving mental and physical stress, especially when coordinated with full, even breathing. We activate the parasympathetic nervous system and its therapeutic capacities through revitalizing backbends, calming standing poses, cooling forward folds, and relaxing restoratives. As you flow through these therapeutic sequences, be present by intentionally scanning the body and noticing how different areas feel—perhaps clenched, tight, sore, or numb. See if you can use your breath to loosen and relax that space. Play with moving in and out of various poses dynamically or holding a shape gently for several breaths and sensing subtle shifts.

Whether you have half an hour for a full sequence or only five minutes to spare, a few key poses you can practice anytime, anywhere are: Wide-legged forward bend (Prasarita Padottanasana), Standing forward bend (Uttanasana), Chest-opener (Anahatasana), Bridge pose (Setu Bandha Sarvangasana), Legs up the wall (Viparita Karani), and Corpse pose (Savasana). We'll explore how these tools calmly energize and release mental anguish. Complement your physical yoga with pranayama breathing and meditation for enhanced effects. Let's examine some anxiety-soothing sequences...

Calming Standing Poses Flow
From Tadasana mountain pose, inhale arms up and gently backbend. Exhale, sweeping arms down by sides, folding into Uttanasana. Bend knees, place hands under feet, and inhale. Straighten legs coming into a flat back. Exhale, step right foot back then left for plank pose. Keep engaging core, and press shoulders away from ears. Inhale, lowering halfway down, exhale, and press back up into the plank. Repeat two more times. Inhale right foot forward, then left, returning into forward fold. Release the torso over the legs, the head hanging heavily. Bend knees deeply, wrap arms under legs and inhale, lift the chest, and straighten legs coming up to stand. Exhale palms together at the heart center. Repeat the second side, starting by back bending arms up. Complete three times on each side with breath.

Next, come into Prasarita Padottanasana with feet wider than hips and toes slightly in. Inhale, lengthen the spine. Exhale, fold forward, placing hands, head, and heart down towards the earth. With each inhale, lengthen the spine forward, and with each exhale release deeper into the forward fold. Hold for 5-8 breaths. Inhale rises back up with a long front torso. Exhale hands to the heart center. Repeat series two more rounds, with three cycles of breath in Prasarita.

Finish by stepping right foot about 12 inches towards the left, coming into the Anahatasana preparatory pose. Lean torso slightly over front leg, grounding back heel. Lift chest towards the sky on inhale, hands interlaced behind back. Exhale folds deeper over the front leg, lowering the chest and head like a pendulum swinging down. Repeat the Anahatasana chest opener five times with breath on each side. Return to Tadasana mountain pose. Close eyes and sense effects.

Soothing Backbend Sequence
From tabletop position, wrists under shoulders, knees under hips - inhale, lift chest forward and up into anahatasana chest expansion. Exhale lower back into the tabletop. Repeat five rounds with breath. Next, curl your toes under, inhale, and lift your knees, hovering in a plank pose. Exhale knees down and untuck toes for child's pose, resting hips on heels. Take 5-8 breaths here, feeling abdomen expand against thighs on inhale, engage the core, drawing navel towards spine upon exhale.

Inhale, come forward onto hands and knees. Exhale cat-cow pose - drop belly lift gaze for cow, arch back round belly for cat - feeling spinal movement mobilizing tension. Repeat cat-cow five times with breath. From all fours, tuck toes, inhale, lift knees hover in plank. Exhale lower down to belly palms by ribs for sphinx pose - chest lifts, gaze forward. Hold the sphinx for five full breaths. Press palms down, lift chest and thighs up for locust pose, engaging glutes and low back. Hold locust five breaths then lower back to belly, turn head to one side for a breath. Switch sides. Lift hips for bow pose - reaching back to grab ankles, gaze forward lifting heart while quadriceps engage. Feel the abdominal stretch. Hold bow pose for five breaths then gently release lying prone.

For counterpose lift the upper body as you slide arms forward, coming onto forearms. Interlace fingers press forearms down, firming shoulder blades together in Sphinx variation. Feel chest expanding on inhales, engage core drawing low belly towards the spine on exhales preventing overarching low back. Hold five breaths. Press up, slide palms forward, lift chest up and back into Anahatasana on all fours - again opening heart center on inhales, drawing naval down towards earth exhales. Repeat anahatasana for five rounds with breath.

Make your way back into tabletop wrists under shoulders, knees under hips. Walk hands a few inches forward of shoulders, curl toes under. Inhale, lift your knees and straighten your legs for a downward-facing dog. Pedal out heels towards mat bending one knee then the other to release low back. Exhale heels press towards the floor. Hold downward dog for five full cycles of breath. Inhale, lift right leg keeping hips square. Open hip for a breath then exhale, step foot forward, lowering left knee down for a low lunge. Press through right foot and straighten back leg for high lunge lifting arms on inhale - opening chest and shoulder girdle. Exhale cartwheel arms down planting palms, and step right foot back into the plank. Hold plank five breaths. Exhale lower to belly, turn head right palms by shoulders for a locust twisting pose. Lift chest thighs, gaze to left, holding five breaths. Gently release prone - turn head to center, take a breath with hands by ribs. Repeat the second side-stepping left foot forward for a low, then high lunge. Hold five breaths, arms overhead, straightening the front leg. Exhale hands down, step left foot back for plank. Hold five breaths. Lower to the floor, turn head left, and lift chest right for twisting locust five breaths. Release down, breath at the center.

A Mindful Path

From a prone position, slide palms underneath the shoulders, press into the tops of the feet, and lift the chest, keeping hips, and legs long for the cobra pose. Engage quads without squeezing your glutes to protect your lower back. Inhale, lift your chest and gaze forward. Exhale release to prone transition up into all fours tabletop position. From tabletop tuck toes under inhale, lift knees, straighten legs press hips up and back for down dog. Exhale, walk feet towards hands for standing forward and fold uttanasana. Release head and torso towards legs. Soften knees as needed. Inhale flat back, look forward, step left foot back, then right, coming into plank pose. Exhale lower to floor pointing toes coming into floor bow pose. Release feet to the floor with knees bent. Inhale rolling over shoulders and press up and back for bridge pose. Lift hips towards the sky. Hold for five breaths. Exhale vertebrae by vertebrae release down. Hug your knees into your chest and give some love to your lower back.

Take the bridge pose again, this time interlacing fingers underneath the body for added lift. Press evenly through shoulders and feet, lifting hips skyward. Draw thighs parallel, open heart to the sky. Stay for five breaths. Exhale release down, and hug your knees in towards your chest. Gently rock side to side, massaging the spine. Draw figure eight with knees loosening up hips. Hug both knees into your chest, straighten your right leg, release your left shin parallel to the floor in half, and do a happy baby pose. Exhale draw left knee back to chest, and straighten right leg. Continue gently rocking, elongating one leg at a time. Or stay with each leg extended for a few breaths. Finish both knees into the chest. Set feet down for final bridge pose - lifting clasping hands underneath press palms down firm shoulder blades as you lift your hips high. Stay five more rounds of breath. Exhale release vertebrae by vertebrae, and hug knees back into the torso letting the spine decompress after soaring skyward. There are a few more gentle rocks side to side if that feels soothing to the spine.

Continue with hugging knees, rocking gently into final release lying flat onto back palms facing up knees together heart centre for Savasana. Close eyes let the body integrate back bending heart and hip opening practice. Sense effects from a deeply calming sequence designed to relieve emotional anxiety and mental overactivity through its physically centering yet expansively uplifting form. Notice sensations from the crown of the head to the tips of the toes. Observe if muscles that felt tense before now seem relaxed. Soften face, relinquishing any residual strain across delicate features. Surrender fully feeling supported not just by the floor beneath you but the vast sky above as well. Spacious cosmos envelop you with infinite understanding and unconditional love. Know that through a commitment to your inner peace profound transformation happens gently with time, organically unveiling layers of luminous tranquility from within rather than chasing anxious thoughts that previously obscured realities of peace lying closer than breath itself - which we return to now during Savasana integrating revitalizing backbends slowly yet steadily cultivating emotional balance breath by breath - steadying turbulent mind as the body settles calmly into its natural openhearted wisdom grounded securely here and now. Honor inner stillness. When ready to close practice gently wiggle fingers and toes, reach arms overhead, and full body stretch. Soft knees roll to your right side pausing briefly. Press up to sit, getting grounded once more. Close eyes bring hands prayer at heart, sending gratitude inward for inner peace practice reveals when you consciously commit to presenting wounds with compassion, not criticism - for critic cannot heal critic. Thus, with self-forgiveness, we reopen doorways to inner calm. Bowhead towards the heart in closing. Namaste.

When the breath wanders, the mind wanders. It is natural for attention to get distracted even during therapeutic movement. Don't judge, just patiently guide your focus back to the sensation of breathing. Like training a wild horse, persistence and kindness work best. With regular practice, attention strengthens - just as muscles support with progressive training adapting in response to steady stimuli. Daily, even brief yoga sessions cultivate mental muscle memory reinforcing relaxation response versus reactive states of stress. In time, we construct graceful inner architecture so responding to life's frictions we meet adversity with steady ease not strain. This liberating neuroplasticity through yoga's alchemy transforms the once restless mind into a reliable refuge. When we commit to inner peace, outer circumstances lose grip - for an untrained mind believes falsehood it needs certain conditions to be happy. Awakened we see no one circumstance grants lasting contentment. Through self-mastery, life unfolds more harmoniously. Daily practice fortifies us with patience and compassion.

Pranayama Practices for Calming Anxiety and Overthinking

The breath is a powerful gateway for addressing anxiety and depression holistically. The yogic theory states that by regulating the breath, you can soothe emotional disturbance, calm mental chatter, and induce deep states of relaxation by activating the parasympathetic nervous system. When we feel anxious or worried, caught in repetitive thought loops, our fight-flight sympathetic activation is heightened. By consciously lengthening exhalations to stimulate the rest-digest physiological response, we quell nervous system arousal, calming the body and mind. Breathwork also increases vitality, mental clarity, emotional resilience, and spiritual insight when practiced regularly.

You can practice pranayama breathing exercises as a seamless part of yoga postures for integrated movement and breathwork, in standalone sessions to quickly relieve stress anytime, or as a moving seated practice coordinated with natural environments for a walking breath meditation outdoors through nature's rejuvenating rhythms and sights. Pair breathwork with meditations for enhanced centering effects, quieting a turbulent mind. Let's explore basic techniques and practical anxiety-relieving sequences...

Simple Calming Pranayama Practices

Equal Breath - Sama Vritti (Sam-ah-vri-tee) – This fundamental yogic breath establishes an even inhalation-exhalation ratio without straining. Sit comfortably with a spine lengthened. Relax shoulders without collapsing chest. Close eyes with chin slightly down. Breathe through the nose unless congested. Focus on smooth, steady breath, conscious yet comfortable. Silently count equal length for the inhale-exhale. Start with a ratio of 4 counts each lasting several seconds for basic pranayama breathing. 5:5 and 6:6 counts work too. Sense abdomen naturally expanding on inhales, drawing gently back on exhales. As you regulate breath consciously notice mental distractions dissipating while clarity and calm increase. After a minute gently release counting breaths. Continue smoothly conscious inhales and exhales a few minutes into the integration phase without force. Finish by taking a rejuvenating full-body stretch, opening your eyes when ready. Equal breaths are very centering and balancing. Practice daily. Advance the ratio slowly, not to strain. Soft belly, steady pacing.

Victorious Breath – Ujjayi (Oo-jai-yee) – Often called Ocean Breath, Ujjayi creates an audible wave-like sound as we breathe consciously through the nose. It helps focus awareness while inducing deep states of calm relaxation for relieving anxiety, and soothing repetitive worrying thoughts and emotional distress generally. Sit comfortably erect yet relaxed. Inhale and exhale fully to open the breathing channels. Exhaling makes a smooth HA sound from the back of the throat like fogging up a mirror. Once you establish the soft throaty HA sound keep it steady for the entire exhale through the nose. Inhale consciously through the nose preferably with the same textured feel at the back of the throat, but without forcing restrictive sensation. Sense expanding abdomen rising with breath filling torso on inhales while exhales feel abdomen gently drawing back towards spine in natural contraction. Close eyes and continue deep conscious Ujjayi for a few minutes then gently release back to normal breathing before finishing with body stretch reenergizing circulation. With practice, the oceanic breath flows smooth and wave-like, calming emotional storms and dissipating mental clouds drifting away. The great relief of anxiety, insomnia, and racing thoughts uplifts depressive moods through conscious yogic breathing.

Breath Counting - Anapanasati (An-uh-pan-uh-suh-tee) – A classic Buddhist meditation for concentrating the ever-wandering mind using the breath as a steady anchor amidst disruptive thought waves. It helps build mental focus, reducing anxiety through breath mindfulness. Sit comfortably yet alert. Gently close your eyes and relax your body without slouching. Inhale consciously counting a silent ONE. Exhale consciously aware of breathing counting silent TWO. Inhale THREE. Exhale FOUR. Count incrementally up to eight with full inhalations-exhalations then simply start again. When the mind loses focus, patiently begin at one again without self-judgment whenever attention drifts into planning, reminiscing, or fantasy. Commit to present moment breath after calming breath. If struggling, stay at lower breath counts before advancing higher. With regular practice mental endurance strengthens, attention stabilizes, and the body relaxes profoundly. After a few minutes gently release the counting technique and just observe natural (encountered) breath until it feels time to finish. Take an energizing full body stretch, opening your eyes and coming back to the external world with calm clarity. Anapanasati breath counting builds attentive focus reducing anxiety and relieves depressive rumination (looping on past/future) through keeping awareness grounded with breath rhythms right here, right now.

Soothing Pranayama Sequence for Calming Anxiety – Sama Vritti, Ujjayi, Viloma

Find a comfortable seat either cross-legged or kneeling on a cushion if needed to ensure knees hover slightly below hips for stability. Lengthen the spine and relax shoulders with no grasping in the neck or effort across the face which remains soft. Allow hands to gently drape on thighs palms facing up in receptive mudra or form Chin or Chinmaya mudra interlacing thumb with index finger near heart center with palms facing up resting on knees which centers energy while invoking grace and wisdom. The tip of the tongue presses gently on the palate connecting the energy circuit for interiority. Close eyes with chin dipped slightly to relax the throat and turn awareness within. Settle into a few minutes of diaphragmatic belly breathing, allowing inhalations to gently fill the rib cage while raising the low belly which recedes back on full, unforced exhalations. Sense centering effects of consciously presencing breath while the body settles and thoughts subside. When ready transition into sama vritti equalizing inhalation-exhalation cycles. Silently begin counting the length of each phase building concentration - inhale FOUR, exhale FOUR - matching duration without strain. Continue equal breath silently counting the ratio of your choice where both inhale-exhale are the same counts. After

Breathing by conscious breath, we steadily redirect attention inward whenever it drifts astray. In time concentration strengthens, and mental endurance for present-moment focus builds. With patient repetition, the tendency to indulge in disruptive thoughts loses grip while breath-awareness stabilizes emotionally calming turbulence within. Sensations and mental scenarios may arise; gently acknowledge them without suppressing or solidifying them. Allow each breath to return focus to the here and now patiently.

After a few minutes of consciously releasing structured breathing technique, continue observing natural inhales and exhales without control just sensory awareness - air gently fills the rib cage on inhales, recedes on exhales as low belly softly compresses. Silently sense breath's soothing rhythm. When ready to close meditation, affirm positive qualities desired for further cultivating through practice - perhaps repeating words like calm, ease, patience, and compassion. Offer self-encouragement to meet what difficulties arise with stability rather than engage in worrying, overthinking or self-criticism which cannot grant peace. To bring palms together alongside the heart center bowing head gently towards hands saying "Namaste " honoring the inner light the practice reveals when committed with courage, not casualness. Take time before opening your eyes to make the transition gradual.

Yoga tools for managing anxiety through movement, breathwork, and meditation help repattern our physiological stress reactions into healthy resilience -- strengthening and soothing the nervous system, stabilizing mood, focusing the mind, and compassionately befriending ourselves amidst emotional storm life brings rather than identifying with each passing weather pattern as solid unchanging reality. By consciously presenting turmoil when it arises, we transmute its contracts into compassionate wisdom, and inner freedom where no condition or circumstance fully dictates happiness. Through dedicating days to wellbeing old wounds heal. At the same time, steady inner peace unfolds - not some flashy peak experience but a humble way of being unperturbed by that which previously knocked us off center. Ancient yogic sciences time-tested and neuroscience confirmed through consistent practice that human consciousness has the power to rewrite our reactions, consciously directing destiny and determining identity no longer hostage to past pain or future worry but liberated into each moment's potential for awakening unconditioned inner joy accessible here and now.

While yoga tools uplift spirits temporarily through each dedication, sustaining antidepressive effects takes committed practice over time gradually rewiring reactive nervous system patterns into resilient new baselines where equanimity becomes a natural response, not a mere ideal. By consciously breathing, moving, and meditating daily we steady wayward attention, encouraging neuroplasticity, making easy and elevated base states more habitual versus effortful. People commonly make New Year's resolutions to get fit yet quickly abandon goals when reactive patterns override inspiring visions unless consciously reinforced through steadfast practice over time fortifying feeble intentions into firm capabilities unable tossed by turbulent tides. While medication may help stabilize biochemistry, enabling one to train steadier, yogic tools heal holistically without side effects, giving agency, kindling our inner healer who wakes to realize their light shines bright enough to dissolve shadows of anxiety and darkness of depression - if boldly honored daily not doctored occasionally.

The courageous path of self-mastery through yoga leads one from restlessness into stillness, isolation to belonging, and helpless suffering into empowered overcoming. By committing precious days to one's liberation, we nurture natural health so innate to living organisms when aligned to rhythms that sustain rather than disrupt life's fundamental flow state. For millennia, householders and sages alike have woven wellness into day's fabric beyond mere medicine but proactive uplifting lifestyle-orienting activities around harmony with nature's organic intelligence manifest as cycles of seasons, cycles of breath, of bassline neurochemical rhythms that organize energy for peak creative expression. Conscious movement, nourishing meals, heartful communion, and meditation's stillness structure schedule not out of rigid legalism but flexible integration valuing health and inner peace no longer relegated disposable when so essentially linked to purposeful living. We transcend limited notions of exercise duration, regimented diets, or seated sessions towards holistic orientation valuing vitality, adaptability, conscious presence, and compassionate wisdom as optimal being's cornerstones.

While intensive training over weeks in an ashram-type setting offers powerful healing results through immersion in retreating from stressful environments, daily practice sustains awakening, stabilizing peace beyond silence into the marketplace of noise, pressure, and turbulence. By dedicating days not weeks to self-mastery, we gradually change our lifestyle's rhythm realigning to healthier harmonic patterns, lifting energy, and outlook, and overcoming momentum. Vibrational medicine restoring resilient flow states helps anxious and depressed surrender striving into being, find grace not gripping, and belong beyond isolation's illusion held by the ego's incessant worries. Through yoga, we remember our inherent completeness no matter the circumstance. Each present moment we inhabit is whole, holy.

Over long expanses, heartfulness becomes boundless. Harmony grows naturally as a garden bed nurturing through patient seasons' ever-blossoming beauty. By learning life's secret, abiding in the present victory reveals from momentary defeats life brings to strengthen through trials and errors we swell wise and modest not hardened but supple souls courageous enough to care. We abandon the anxious chase of misplaced dreams that never satisfy by presenting eternal wellsprings close as this breath awaiting awareness of abundance within. We transmute depressive pasts rooted in loss or abuse by compassionately holding this moment conscious it will pass without solidifying reactions. Equanimity stabilizes seeing phenomena as cloud patterns pass. This too, shall change and become a hopeful slogan calming turbulence. We breathe blessings out to all beings, fortifying universal belonging beyond personal lack. We inhabit eternal now bold enough to bow heads and surrender striving for security into life's mysteries, which open us beyond controlling what was never ours. We free fall through illuminating uncertainty - faith's leap revealing invisible wings as we let go of forces vaster than our comprehending. The smile behind all forms awakens as each inhalation returns awareness to the home where we already belong.

Cultivating Mindfulness and Self-Compassion Through Meditation

While physical postures calm and soothe the body, relieving muscular armoring patterns that manifest from chronic anxiety/depression, seated meditations grant direct access to the mind's tendency to endlessly spin out cascades of thoughts that heighten stress through worrying, planning and judgmental assessments of circumstances, self and others. By training in present-moment attention beyond such mental scenarios projected by the ego-mind, we contact subtler dimensions of the inner terrain revealing naturally tranquil awareness unperturbed by passing storms of adversity or emotion. Neuroscience confirms meditation literally transforms our stress responses long term, cultivating an observant equanimity and compassion that easily accommodates any experience without suppression or over-identifying with temporary conditions.

As American Buddhist nun Pema Chodron conveyed: Meditation helps us develop a tender heart endowed with courage. By stabilizing attention beyond the ego-mind's incessant commentary, we grow friendly towards all aspects of our human experience - even difficult emotions and pain held consciously lose their binding powers over identity otherwise experienced as solid, oppressively real. Like dark thunderclouds passing through the vast sky, sensations arise and dissolve ever-changing; by anchoring in the still space of pure awareness, all-weather moves through this permeable presence without disturbing peaceful embodiment unconditionally as the atmosphere receives all activity within its embrace.

While physical postures unwind bodily holding patterns that manifest anxiety/depression somatically, seated meditation grants access to the mind's tendency to endlessly spin out thoughts that heighten stress through future worrying and judgmental assessments within or about external situations. By patiently training present-moment attention beyond the ego-mind's turbulent thought form projections powered by past impressions and karmic propensities, we stabilize awareness in the innately tranquil space of pure consciousness always already available beneath mental storms however emotionally intense at surface levels. In time this awakens practitioners to subtler dimensions of inner terrain revealing natural clarity unconditioned by identities and beliefs previously over-identified with. We relax into enduring awareness like a vast sky unperturbed by passing weather patterns through consciously embedding into this stable ground no matter which direction winds whip.

Neuroscience shows meditation transforms stress responses longterm by strengthening neural pathways of regulation, resilience, and higher perspective-taking beyond habitual reactions. A study from Harvard found that mindful meditators consciously process emotions without suppressing yet also avoiding over-identifying via narrative spin habitually attached to challenging feeling states. Equanimity accompanies compassion. Present-moment attention stabilizes reflexivity, empowering calmer choices aligned to values not just impulses. Researchers discovered not only immediate but accumulating and enduring changes in receptor density, gray matter volumes, and amygdala reactions in regions related to meta-cognition, body awareness, and empathy. This confirms experiential relief from afflicted mental states into enlightened meaning-making, radical acceptance, and self-compassion through techniques neurologically building stress resilience capacities with practice.

Ancient meditative disciplines East to West centralize slowing and deepening breath while concentrating attention faculties one-pointedly on an object like a flame or phrase. This stabilizes awareness from excessive scattering that renders perception chaotic and identity confused, helping recollect dispersed energies wasted worrying, planning, remembering/regretting what no longer serves. Modern teachers incorporate these contemplative sciences into contemporary contexts using breath, sound, or bodily regions of focus conveying creative visualization and compassion meditations. Whether following structured sequences or sitting supportively witnessing mental/emotional patterns arise and pass trusting intrinsic awareness will organically settle and clear; we cultivate non-reactive space for the turmoil to move through experience without gaining a foothold as a solid oppressed reality. By granting unconditional loving presence we alchemize suffering's binding force through courageously feeling without fixating on negative narratives that previously perpetuated disturbances. Equanimity stabilizes unconditionally by passing phenomena. We inhabit eternal now, bold enough to bow heads and surrender striving for security into life's great mysteries which cannot help but open us.

The fruits of dedication to meditation's path convey non-conceptual inner belonging beyond longing, steady well-being not contingent on sensorial highs, lovingly allowing all experience while relinquishing the habitual need to control life's fundamentally unpredictable and ephemeral essence. By consciously embedding into the sacred ground of now, practitioners stabilize compassionate non-dual perception gracefully including apparent polarities and paradoxes of relative reality into integral evolutionary worldview interbeing with others as divine expressions of primordial awareness itself - the I AM-ness accessible when thought interpretations that divide cease. This culminates in enduring spiritual freedom no matter the ups and downs. We relax as love into the uncertainty, rooted in unborn unmade, undying.

Prof. Mark Fanning

Chapter 7

Building Resilience Through Pranayama and Pratyahara

Exploring Pranayama Breathing Techniques

As we explored in earlier chapters, prana refers to the vital life force energy that runs through and animates all living beings. Pranayama is the practice of controlling the breath to work with this essential life energy. Through conscious breathing techniques, we can circulate prana to every cell of the body and mind, energizing our being, calming emotional storms, and cultivating greater resilience to life's inevitable ups and downs.

Patanjali describes pranayama as a method of steadying the mind's fluctuations. When we feel stressed or anxious, our breath reflects that inner state, becoming short, shallow, and uneven. By consciously working with the breath, however, we can break this stress feedback cycle and facilitate deeper states of calm, clarity, and insight. As Paramahansa Yogananda once affirmed, "Breath has sound, rhythm, and depth. It creates and activates certain centers in the human body, causing them to vibrate. The science of breath was and still is taught by all great yoga masters to stabilize body, breath, and mind." Across yoga's history, practices such as Alternate Nostril Breathing, Ujjayi Pranayama, and Cooling Breath have been transmitted as tools for relieving mental turbulence and returning to stability amid life's storms. Yet, to harness their benefits, we must first understand the basics.

The full yogic breath employs the entire respiratory capacity by leveraging the diaphragm and intercostal muscles surrounding the rib cage. It thus stands in contrast to the shallow chest breathing many of us unconsciously carry out. To experience this fuller breath...

Applying Pratyahara to Turn Inward

As we regulate the breath through pranayama, we also begin minimizing outward sensory disturbances through pratyahara, the fifth limb of yoga. Pratyahara means "withdrawal" or "sensory transcendence." It is the conscious process of internalizing our awareness, and filtering out external stimuli that drain our energies.

Sitting in meditation, we may hear cars honking or construction rumbling outside. The phone might ring, an email might ping, or family members might call our name. Such sensory disruptions scatter the mind as it grasps after external diversions. Pratyahara involves gently disengaging from these stimuli, retaining focus inward.

As an analogy, picture yourself looking out the window of a moving train. Fixating on the flickering scenes, you might feel dizzy or disoriented. Yet by drawing the blind, you close out the visual turbulence. Now gazing ahead into the train car, motion steadies and balance restores. Pratyahara works much the same for the wandering mind. As we stop chasing outward scenes, inner stillness naturally settles.

A Mindful Path

Initially, this turning inward requires conscious effort. Yet, over time, periods of pratyahara unveil our mind's naturally serene depths beneath the choppy surface waves. As pratyahara deepens, we enter profound states of concentration in which we become wholly absorbed in the present. Hours may pass like minutes. Some yogic traditions describe this as turiya, the fourth state beyond waking, dreaming, and deep sleep. Modern psychologists call it "flow".

Athletes know this as "the zone," musicians as "feeling the groove," and artists as "losing themselves in the creative flow." Time blinks off; distractions dissolve, and inspiration erupts. This optimal flow emerges from sustained pratyahara, filtering sensory disruptions while sustaining focus. Bursts of genius or bliss bubble up from unconscious realms unimpeded by the rational mind's constraints. We touch eternal witness consciousness, detached from external worries.

While such peak performance moments appear rare for most, the yogic journey reveals this witnessing awareness as our essential nature beneath passing storms. Meditators describe pratyahara as "settling into being" or "coming home." There remains much to do but nowhere to go. We rest as unbounded awareness itself, liberated from all efforts to be different, better, or other than we already are.

Yet this inner homecoming requires training the puppy mind not to run outward each moment it gets compulsively. So, we diligently practice returning attention again and again to an interior anchor. This develops the mind's ability to choose where it directs awareness rather than living at the mercy of passing impulses. As intention overrides impulsion, we gain access to deeper dimensions of stillness. Inner transformation unfolds.

Prof. Mark Fanning

While physical postures realign the gross physical structure, subtle yogic techniques targeting the nervous system and energy body cultivate mental and emotional resilience transcending crisis reactivity. Originating before complex asanas emerged, pranayama breathing exercises and sensory withdrawal practices rapidly recalibrate mind-body homeostasis. Building a regular foundation with these portable, low-effort yet high-yield tools empowers maintaining inner peace amidst outer turmoil.

As the interface between body and mind, the breath proves an extremely effective leverage point for self-regulation. By consciously harnessing the power of this automatic process, pranayama rapidly overrides dysfunctional activation patterns. Deep rhythmic breathing signals safety to the nervous system, reducing fight-or-flight reactions. Increasing respiratory stamina and efficiency through practices like ocean breath and bellows breath optimizes energy available for higher executive functions. As the body mindfully settles, mental distress similarly clears. Lightness pervades consciousness once constrictions are released.

However, the untrained often underestimate the risks of improperly practicing intense breathing techniques without proper education. Trying excess external breath retention absent extensive lung capacity strains the system rather than uplifting vitality. Additionally, loud vocalized breathing performs catharsis yet requires responsibility to channel released energies constructively. Begin with softer approaches, truly calming the nervous system before incorporating advanced practices. Start where you are even if simply observing normal breathing rhythms. Then, gradually extend inhalations and exhalations building tolerance.

The sister's practice of supporting pranayama develops pratyahara, withdrawal of outgoing sensory engagement, and calming stimulation-seeking impulses. Pratyahara employs specific sensory channel purification exercises, teaching students how to consciously dial up or down specific sights, sounds, tastes, textures and smells flooding consciousness. Bodily scanning practices similar to yoga nidra attune felt senses of inner vibration and flow even in stillness. As sensory grasping relaxes, the mental grip on desires similarly releases allowing non-attached equanimity and higher insight.

With roots of obsessiveness or overstimulation revealed through this inner examination, students release tight mental grasping towards destructive thought loops. Balance restores attention bias away from stimulus hunger towards inner richness, nurturing natural vitality. Demonstrations of pratyahara advanced students even demonstrate conscious control of autonomic processes like stopping the heart or altering skin temperature using the mind as a scalpel into neurology. But beginner steps allow safe exploration of inner terrain where sensory experience merges into energetic awareness.

While pranayama and pratyahara elicit immediate neurological shifts, developing mastery sustains the emotional resilience necessary for weathering inevitable life storms. Consistent practice builds capacity similar to physical muscle memory. The more we consciously relax under pressure, the more this self-regulation strategy stabilizes as a default response.

Certain pranayama ratios balance sympathetic exhilaration with parasympathetic renewal. For example, lengthening the exhalation triggers relaxation while extended inhalation energizes. Balancing these solar and lunar breaths prevents burnout from chronic stress. The ratio of 4:6:8 counting regulates heart rate variability, signaling systemic coherence. Combining breathing exercises with mudras and bandhas further roots conscious access to normally involuntary processes.

Prof. Mark Fanning

Many techniques bridge pratyahara sensory withdrawal with concentration. Trataka candle gazing stills visual restlessness while observing the afterimage strengthens retractive skills. Alternate nostril breathing similarly purifies latent karma clouding mental clarity to access deeper wisdom. Other pratyahara methods employ mantra repetition, visualization of inner energy centers, or alchemical purification of elemental essences animating consciousness.

Over time, these skills allow conscious control over fight, flight, or freeze reactivity programmed through trauma but now updated through presence. Neither repressing nor indulging compulsive habits, we retain compassionate inner freedom to choose higher functioning aligned with deeper values. When destructive impulses unravel under conscious investigation, our intrinsic goodness naturally flowers in its place.

On the highest level, mastery of pranayama and pratyahara prepares consciousness for unity beyond all opposites. No longer identifying with passing phenomena builds meditative witness embodiment. By continually relaxing rather than grasping towards any sensation, eternal bliss increasingly emerges as our essential nature. Since external happiness inevitably fluctuates, inner joy remains unshakeable once established. We come to trust transcendental equanimity overtaking consciousness whenever we stop judging the moment. In absolute stillness, reveal the peaceful awareness containing all creation dreaming existence into being.

84

Chapter 8

Yoga Nidra and Deep Relaxation: Restoring Inner Harmony

Yoga Nidra: Gateway to Deep Relaxation

Yoga Nidra is an ancient meditation practice that guides one into a state of profound relaxation. In this unique state, the body is at complete rest while the mind remains awake and inwardly aware. For centuries, yogis have used this technique to reduce tension, regulate emotional imbalance, and tap into deeper aspects of consciousness.

The term "Yoga Nidra" comes from two Sanskrit words, yoga meaning "union or one-pointed awareness" and Nidra meaning "sleep." However, Yoga Nidra is very different from normal sleep; it creates changes in brain wave patterns, allowing access to 'hypnagogic' states normally experienced only as we fall asleep or wake up. But with training and guidance, we can remain alert and conscious during Yoga Nidra to receive its full benefits.

During a session, a teacher verbally guides the practitioner through four main stages: internalization, Sankalpa, rotation of consciousness, and ending the practice. This systematic methodology brings about a definite shift from beta brain waves that dominate our normal waking state to slower alpha, theta, and delta waves. This induces full-body relaxation while sustaining awareness. Let's explore what unfolds in each stage of this unique meditative therapy.

Stage 1: Internalization

The first stage turns one's attention fully inward to disconnect from the external environment. To begin, the teacher instructs students to come into Savasana or Corpse Pose, lying flat on their backs without crossed limbs. With the body settled and eyes closed, the mind too can withdraw focus from sights, sounds, and physical sensations happening around us.

As one directs attention inside, the guiding voice becomes the only auditory input. Streamlining sensory stimuli helps concentration zoom inward to arise centered between the eyebrows. This interiorized attention is called pratyahara, described as the fifth limb of classical Ashtanga Yoga. Withdrawing the usual scatter of senses, thoughts, and disturbances forms an intentioned act of dissociation from the outside world.

Having detached from inputs inviting mental commentary, the restless consciousness gets an opportunity to direct attention where we choose. In Yoga Nidra, we take one-pointed awareness first to different bodily regions and then deep into subtle energies behind all mental fluctuations. This internalization shift brings tangible relief from an overloaded nervous system, letting the somatic burdens carried from worldly involvement now simply fall away.

Stage 2: Sankalpa

Having arrived centered inside one's own experience, the second stage involves setting a Sankalpa - a firm personal intention stated during the practice. The teacher invites students to reflect, and then clearly declare an objective they wish to strengthen or manifest through their Yoga Nidra practice.

A Sankalpa functions as a seed planted in the fertile soil of the subconscious mind. This seed can sprout and grow into embodied experience or conscious realization when properly cared for. Intuitive wisdom reveals that energetic potentials - whether constructive or destructive - must first exist in the mental sphere before crystallizing into external realities over time. Yoga Nidra allows you to consciously hone and amplify chosen potentials so they structure life experiences aligned to your highest purpose.

When setting your aspiration, phrase the Sankalpa in simple present tense as if it's already unfolding. This positive language mirrors an outcome already achieved that you now step into energetically. The classic template is: "I am ______" filling the blank with the change wished for like improved health, diminished anxiety, enhanced creativity, or loving relationships. State it with clarity and heartfelt focus up to seven times, allowing the meaning to reverberate through all layers of your psyche.

Once clearly set, let the Sankalpa go to work silently and indirectly on your behalf. There's no need to clutch it desperately as the conscious ego often does with goals. Simply plant the seed of your heart's longing then relax back, trusting life's inherent intelligence to orchestrate the natural fruition in proper timing. Of course, growth depends partly on environmental conditions, too. So between Yoga Nidra sessions, act as a humble gardener carefully nurturing healthy soil through self-inquiry, lifestyle regimens, or removing inner obstacles as they arise.

While asana poses and pranayama breathing rectifies muscular tension and restless thought patterns, yoga nidra deep relaxation elicits even more profound systemic recalibration. By effortlessly sinking the thinking mind into lower brainwave states, yoga nidra allows full-spectrum reset reorganizing neurological, metabolic, and subtle energetic pathways fueling consciousness. Regularly returning to this inner sanctuary of tranquility ensures lasting integration of higher states realized during active meditation.

The simple ritual of yoga nidra efficiently guides even beginners through integrative phases of internalization, settling, grounding and uplifting. First, turning attention away from the outer world removes overstimulating sensory input. Initial body scans next unravel residual muscular, respiratory, and psychological tension. As the system unwinds, consciousness sinking into deeper beings balances stimulation and exciting sympathetic fight-or-flight nerves with parasympathetic rest-and-digest relaxation.

With the stage set through withdrawal and release, specific nidra techniques can target localized tension or imbalances. Visualizations, affirmations, and resolutions subsequently reprogram neuromuscular wiring, transform negative emotional patterns, and solidify desired intentions at the subconscious level. Finally emerging realigns body, breath, and mind to embody elevated baselines throughout daily activity. Over time, this alchemy balances energy expenditure with renewal, restoring holistic well-being.

The healing effects of deep relaxation concentrate pratyahara's sensory withdrawal inward for systemic homeostasis. Physiologically, metabolic processes restore optimal functioning depleted by chronic stress. Lymphatic flow accelerates waste removal while hormone levels linked to resilience like oxytocin and endogenous endorphins replenish. Nerves fire more efficiently, and genome expression favors growth and repair. Psychologically, yoga nidra facilitates the integration of daily experiences, allowing the emergence of insight, inspiration, and maturity.

Subtly, yoga nidra repairs gaps or blockages within the energy body damaged by traumatic experience or neglect. Skipping this phase of self-recovery risks Energetic leaks accumulated over years until pathologies manifest physically or psychologically. That is why yogic living emphasizes daily renewal rituals. Regular realignment prevents energy deficits demanding crisis intervention down the line when disease advances. Think of yoga nidra as closing energetic cycles opcncd during productive yet depleting daily activities.

The deep tranquility permeating consciousness during yoga nidra gives access to elevated dimensions of awareness inaccessible to the thinking mind. Subtle impressions and latent intentions held in somatic memory arise at the surface of conscious articulation. By tracking the interconnection of sensations, images, feelings and intuitions, new holistic coherence integrates fragmented aspects of self.

This consolidation process rewires self-concepts, decision-making structures, and even cellular biology towards unity. Yogis consider the bashful state-induced balancing and unifying opposite hemispheres of the brain, subtle energy channels, and nervous system domains. Resolutions set here bypass mental constructs and limiting beliefs otherwise obstructing conscious potential. Aligned integrity of body, energy, and soul calibrates the bio-computer towards optimal performance.

While even brief yoga nidra sessions offer immense therapeutic value, longer guided journeys allow fuller psychological integration within unmanifest realms of being. The traditional eight-limb sequence moves systematically through the innermost levels from gross physiology towards increasingly subtle aspects of energetic, emotional, and spiritual embodiment. We witness universal polarities like chaos and order, fear and love, death and birth. Exploring the gradients between these apparent opposites unifies their essence beyond the intellect.

This non-conceptual landscape of pure feeling reconciles fragmented emotions and memories. By welcoming disowned shadow aspects back home into conscious identity, they no longer control behavior unconsciously. We uncover boundless inner space unaffected by life's passing storms. Every sensation mirrors universal processes flowing through the timeless Self non-separate from transcendental awareness underneath passing phenomena. Ultimately chambers of the heart reopen to selfless compassion towards all beings.

While difficult to grok cognitively, regular conscious deep dive adventures build embodied familiarity with yoga nidra's transcendent yet immanent inner sanctuary of stillness. Maintaining a connection to this insulated oasis empowers maintaining equilibrium amidst the rollercoaster of daily life. No matter what mental, emotional, or external challenges you face, this inner resource of renewed potential remains untouched yet readily available once again. By simply relaxing into being, ultimate soul freedom reveals itself here and now as your natural state beyond all states.

Prof. Mark Fanning

Chapter 9

Integrating Yoga Wisdom into Modern Mental Healthcare

Understanding the Mind-Body Connection in Yoga

Yoga is an ancient system of health and wellbeing that recognizes the deep connections between the mind, body, and spirit. Modern science has only recently begun validating what yogic wisdom has asserted for millennia - that our thoughts, emotions, and lifestyle choices profoundly impact our physical and mental health.

In the yoga tradition, the body and mind are seen as two facets of one's larger being rather than separate entities. What affects one aspect affects the whole. When we experience emotional turmoil or prolonged stress, it manifests physically as muscle tension, headaches, digestive issues, or exacerbation of chronic illnesses. When we nurture the body through movement, breathing techniques, and proper nutrition, it has a stabilizing influence on our nervous system and mood.

Yoga offers us tools to break free of harmful thought patterns, balance emotional overwhelm, and ease the body through postures, breathwork, and meditation. Through regular practice, we gain insight into where we hold mental and physical tension to consciously shift into a more balanced, integrated state of being.

The yogic view of the mind challenges common Western notions locating mental function strictly within the cranial space of the brain or skull. While neurobiology illuminates key areas involved in cognition, from the holistic perspective of yoga philosophy, diverse faculties contribute to the broad concept of "mind" in its various expressions. Most foundational is Ahamkara, the faculty generating personal self-identity and willpower. Buddhi describes the higher discerning intellect with abilities to discriminate between ultimate reality and temporary illusion. Manas relates to the lower, restless-thinking mind constantly processing sensory information and emotional reactions. Beyond even subcortical unconscious drives, Chitta represents the deepest storehouse of all conscious and subconscious impressions accumulated through personal and ancestral memory. These various aspects of individual consciousness interoperate dynamically to generate the emergent experience of being "me" navigating internal thoughts, capes, and external environments. By harmonizing these distinct mental forces, the integrated mind harnesses full innate wisdom, clarity, and compassion towards existential liberation from suffering.

Together, these facets create our distinctive mental energy field or psyche. By training these aspects of the mind, we can override old conditioned patterns and establish new supportive neural pathways and habits.

Modern psychology has begun to recognize that besides our rational, thinking brain lies an intelligent "body-mind" with its inherent wisdom. When we are trapped in obsessive thoughts or overwhelming emotions, shifting our attention to physical sensations and movements can calm the nervous system and unlock deeper ways of knowing.

Yoga offers a framework for accessing this innate body-mind intelligence. Through practicing mindful asana sequences, breathing techniques, and meditation, we connect to the body's subtle sensations, energies, and rhythms. As we become more attuned to these quieter signals underlying our conscious thought streams, we gain liberating new perspectives. Rather than being caught up in the churning mental waves, we find a still island at our core - a place of clarity and compassionate witnessing.

Cultivating presence through yoga allows us to objectively observe our thought patterns without judgment. We may come to realize that identifying with each passing thought as absolute truth is flawed. Getting entangled in negative ruminations and stories draws us away from directly contacting the peace and joy that lies beneath the surface. Continually returning body, breath, and mind to the present moment fosters equanimity and inner calm.

As yoga students delve deeper, the emphasis slowly shifts from outer effort and striving towards receptive being and allowing. We intuitively learn where we are tight or imbalanced and how to return to overall equilibrium and wholeness. Rather than aggressively forcing the body or breath into conventional ideas of what they "should" look like, we respect organic limitations and honor the innate rhythms that want to unfold uniquely through us.

This inner work of freeing the body, breath, and mind from restricted movement patterns and limiting beliefs mirrors the process of emotional growth. Releasing long-held tensions and opening up to new ways of feeling, thinking, and responding allows for greater adaptability, resilience, and range of expression.

Prof. Mark Fanning

Yoga provides a comprehensive roadmap for understanding and transforming our habitual energy patterns on the physical, mental, emotional, and spiritual planes. Through diligent self-study both on and off the mat, genuine healing and awakening can unfold.

Cultivating Presence and Mindfulness

The cornerstone of yogic practice is presence—the ability to witness the workings of body and mind with equanimity calmly. When we're fully present, we're not lost in regrets over the past or worries about the future. The practice of mindfulness teaches us to continually return to the here and now, recognizing each moment with fresh eyes.

Modern psychology now recognizes the profound healing effects of living mindfully. Studies show just eight weeks of mindfulness training can structurally change the brain, reducing reactivity to stress. Tuning into the present dilutes the constant mental chatter fueled by fear and uncertainty. We realize many upsetting thoughts and emotions lack substance when viewed objectively. By repeatedly guiding attention to sensations and immediate perceptions, we train the mind to anchor in what is real versus the imagined.

As we scan the body during yoga posture sequences, we cultivate interoceptive awareness. Tuning into subtle breath rhythms and fluctuating energy levels teaches us to detect and release accumulated tensions before they build. If feeling anxious about an event next week, we consciously shift to apprehend the safety and stability of the present moment experience.

Getting caught up in narratives and judgments often amplifies suffering. A mindfulness approach allows us to neutrally label thoughts as "planning," "criticizing," or "worrying" and return to embodied presence. Rather than suppressing unpleasant content, we create space around it. By catching our identification patterns earlier, we strengthen our self-regulatory capacity rather than resorting to impulsive reactions.

The Ethical Framework of Yoga

Beyond techniques for managing stress, classical yoga offers an ethical framework promoting virtues like self-restraint, contentment, and compassion. The primary text of yoga philosophy, The Yoga Sūtras, describes these qualities and practices which encourage stability and peace of mind.

Contentment is viewed as essential for mental equilibrium and growth. When we feel Self-acceptance and gratitude for simple pleasures, we don't depend as much on external conditions for happiness. We can better handle life's curves when not overly attached to one outcome. Learning to pause and truly digest experiences before pursuing the next thing fosters integrity.

Cultivating positive regard and goodwill towards others also alleviates the mind. Helping fellow beings primes neurochemical systems associated with trust and bonding. Reacting with empathy rather than anger transforms relationships. We remember basic goodness resides in everyone when their actions seem hurtful or thoughtless. Holding this expansive perspective uplifts and reminds us of interdependence.

The concept of Mitahara describes the yogic approach to nutrition and healthy consumption. Pursuing wholesome sensory experiences in moderation allows the mind to settle. When we regularly overeat, overshop, overwork, or overindulge in digital entertainment, instability follows. The body-mind loses resilience and agility to adapt swiftly. Yoga teaches consumption habits that impact not just physical health but mental health. Balancing indulgence with self-restraint helps maintain constitutional strength.

Understanding the Mind's Conditioning

Yoga views most emotional suffering as learned conditioning layered upon our original essence of peace and unconditional joy. As infants, we perceive the world without preconceived judgment. Gradually, as neural pathways develop, we acquire filters from societal conditioning and past hurts. Fears form of not having core needs met—for safety, belonging, and self-worth. We adopt coping mechanisms like people-pleasing or hostile withdrawal. By young adulthood subconscious reaction patterns solidify yet keep us stuck responding the same way.

Negative thought loops and entrenched emotional traits feel intrinsic, but yoga suggests they were acquired. Digesting life experiences through a less conditioned mind could have led to vastly different beliefs and self-images. We mistakenly give absolute truth status to perspectives warped by limited awareness and immature resources to process challenges. By recognizing conditioned attitudes as changeable, we reclaim the power to shape an identity aligned with our highest values consciously.

The limbic system and amygdala, central to regulating emotions, stay malleable across the lifespan. We can train different emotional set points by installing supportive beliefs, calming breathing rhythms, and balancing nervous system activation. Meditating on positive qualities we wish to strengthen and reshape neural structure. With consistent reinforcement, new thought patterns and behavior replace reactionary ones formed in childhood or adolescence when we lack clear understanding. Yogic self-transformation requires courage and perseverance yet offers radical freedom.

Understanding the Mind's Layers

Rather than a single unitary entity, yogic philosophy describes separate interacting layers of the mind. The manomaya kosa relates to processing sensory input and concrete thought. Like a software program, it depends on the hardware of the gross物质的 body and nerves to function. However, when we meditate, the mind continues digesting concepts and experiences independent of sensual data. This suggests a subtler mental plane.

The vijñānamaya kosa relates to this deeper faculty evaluating experiences beyond immediate stimuli. It integrates direct perceptions with emotional memories and belief systems in our psychological makeup. Yogis, traveling inward through these layers of consciousness, discovered a blissful silent source from which all minds emerge. Named Chitta in Sanskrit teachings, this universal field stores the archetypal patterns behind all forms in nature. Tuning consciousness into this transcendent yet immanent reality brings intuitive insight and liberation from conditioned identities.

Purifying Negative Emotions

Just as we care for physical health through nutrition and movement, yoga offers specific methods for cleansing toxins from the emotional body. Practices like heart salutation (Anjali Mudra) are performed with conscious breathing to purge sadness, fear, and anger. Flowing vinyasa sequences paired with music FLUSH stuck energies from cells. Alternate nostril breathing (Nadi Shodhana) clears the imbalance between masculine and feminine nervous system channels.

Chanting vibrational mantras as Om washes away subconscious residue still coloring perception.

Once emotional buildup is released through these cleansing rituals, negative reactivity lessens. We embody the philosophical concept of Pratipaksha Bhavana by consciously installing uplifting replacement thoughts. We affirm positive truths about our inherent goodness and connectedness whenever pessimistic mental tapes or emotional looping starts. We continually turn the mind towards the light until the elevation remains steady. Combining asana, pranayama, mantra, and meditation makes transformation stick by reinforcing new neural nets daily

The Peace That Lives Within Us All

While maturing our responses, yoga helps transmute negative emotions themselves into higher potentials. Anger when redirected fuels assertion to set necessary boundaries or advocacy for justice. Fear when harnessed propels proactive planning and preparation. Sadness when allowed passage waters the soil for fresh seeds of meaning and purpose to sprout. Rather than rejecting parts of human experience, yoga offers processes for digesting all of it into wholeness.

Beneath passing storms of thought and emotion, yoga guides us to our spiritual essence—pure undisturbed awareness. Termed Jivatman, it represents the individualized aspect of the infinite Universal Self that breathes through all beings. Realizing experientially this unbroken ground of Being which lies within and connects us all, is considered the pinnacle revelation in yogic wisdom.

A Mindful Path

It takes reflection to recognize outer situations don't deterministically control inner peace. We unwittingly hand away power by making circumstances or other's actions responsible for emotional states. In reality, we don't have to wait for anything external to prove our worth or validate our purpose to feel whole and at ease right now. The liberating secret is happiness always remains within and available regardless of what happens—we simply overlooked its quiet unwavering presence!

What we seek lives already inside us—a deep knowing of our completeness beyond words, concepts, or changing conditions. Yoga gives experiential methods to realize this, not just philosophically understand it intuitively. Once the eyes perceive that inner treasure awaiting all along, old fears and contractions loosen. We relax into the fullness of who we are – what yoga calls one's True Nature or Svabhava. From here compassionate engagement with all of life flows freely.

While pharmaceuticals and psychotherapy remain frontline treatments for most psychiatric disorders, a growing body of research demonstrates yoga's potential as an adjunctive or alternative therapy. An ancient mind-body science predating modern medicine, yoga offers a spectrum of safe, low-cost tools for regulating nervous system imbalance and distorted thought patterns fueling mental health conditions. Integrative clinics now incorporate yoga-based breathing, meditation, and movement techniques to successfully improve outcomes for anxiety, trauma, depression, addiction, eating disorders, psychosis, and more.

However, flawed interpretations of yoga philosophy can inadvertently enable dysfunctional behaviors often driven by underlying psychological wounds or personality disorders. Simply infusing asana with positive mantras fails to address deep-rooted afflictive patterns skillfully. Similarly, pushing through intense pain or breath retention in the name of spiritual growth often aggravates psychological problems. While advanced practices have legitimate therapeutic applications in certain contexts, the untrained often misapply intense catharsis as panacea.

Responsibly leveraging yoga for mental health care, therefore relies on nuanced assessment of appropriate tools calibrated to each student's diagnosis, abilities, and support systems. For example, stimulatory breathing practices used judiciously can alleviate sluggish depression yet may trigger manic episodes in bipolar patients. Cooling Yin therapy stabilizes mania while worsening depressive stagnation. Just as no single pharmaceutical universally applies, individualized yoga therapy considers unique root causes driving disorders.

FOUNDATIONAL LAYER

The most universally accessible starting point integrates gentle somatic practices smoothing out neurological stress activation. Here, simple breathing exercises, mindfulness techniques, and gentle movement dial down fight-or-flight reactivity by lowering cortisol, heart rate, and blood pressure. As the nervous system settles, students gain meta-awareness of ingrained triggers through attentive detachment rather than reflexive identification. Over time, effective self-regulation skills enable responding consciously rather than unconsciously even amidst familiar triggers.

The subtle yogic technology of Pratyahara provides additional leverage for handling sensory input overload comorbid across many diagnoses. Pratyahara employs specific sensory channel purification exercises, teaching students how to consciously dial up or down specific sights, sounds, tastes, textures and smells flooding the nervous system. Developing reflexive sensitivity control empowers self-care strategies long after classes end. With roots of obsessiveness or overstimulation revealed, students release tight grasping to destructive thought loops. Balance restores attention bias towards positivity and prosocial behavior through natural joy.

While foundational practices establish crucial distress tolerance skills, many students also benefit from targeted techniques addressing root psychological and energetic causes of specific conditions. For trauma recovery, gentle somatic experiencing paired with non-verbal creative arts therapies skillfully navigates the activation of traumatic memory imprints locked in the nervous system without re-traumatization. Here, movement rituals help discharge frozen fight, flight, or freeze responses while relational attunement with the therapist redistributes disrupted attachment patterns.

Alternatively, eating disorders driven by an obsession with bodily control find liberation through practices cultivating radical self-acceptance like a meditation on the inner witness consciousness or Divine Light. Anorexia and bulimia often accompany addictive perfectionism rooted in distorted self-concepts and negative self-talk that yogic philosophy exposes as false identities. Here, neti neti inquiry, positive affirmations, mirror work, and chanting shift ingrained self-judgment by unveiling the peaceful whole self beyond mental constructs.

Students suffering from depression, anxiety, and other mood disorders plagued by ruminative thinking additionally utilize concentration and insight techniques, redirecting awareness away from negative narrative loops. Mantra meditation crowds out bottom-up depressive rumination with top-down prefrontal control while vipassana insight practices expose the transient, selfless nature of destructive thought patterns. Over time, metacognition skills enable self-liberation from attachment to stories robbing mental bandwidth. Yogic lifestyle and dietary guidelines also recalibrate biological rhythms and neurotransmitter balance disturbed in mood disorders.

While yoga alone cannot cure serious psychiatric illnesses, this time-tested system empowers psychological self-mastery complementary to conventional treatment. The embodied awareness cultivated through experiential somatic and subtle energy practices ultimately transcends intellectual compliance with healthy habits. Ethically conducted as therapy, ancient sciences offer modern medicine universal tools for sustainability through endogenous bio-psycho-spiritual healing. Instead of mere symptom suppression, yoga targets root existential causes of suffering across all mental health diagnoses. Integrated with compassionate psychotherapy, yoga provides foundational skills and enduring resources for thriving beyond diagnosis.

Chapter 10

Creating a Personal Sadhana: Establishing an Enduring Mind-Body Practice

Exploring Your Intention and Motivation

As we build a personal yoga practice, the first step is turning our attention inward to understand our deepest intentions. Every lasting endeavor starts with the seed of an aspiration that keeps calling us forward. What is calling you to establish a sadhana in your journey? What do you hope to gain or experience through daily yoga practice? Contemplating this can reveal much about what we long for at the core of our being.

For many, the initial draw to yoga comes from a desire for physical strength, flexibility, balance, and grace in the body. Yet embodied practice plants us firmly in the present moment, helping reconnect us to subtler realms of intuition, creativity, peace, and wholeness. As yoga philosopher B.K.S Iyengar expressed, "The body is your temple. Keep it pure and clean for the soul to reside in." Cultivating presence through asana and pranayama lays the foundation for personal transformation on many levels.

Others come seeking relief from anxiety, depression, trauma, or simply the stress of modern life. Yoga promises a refuge from mental turbulence, but its gifts encompass far more. A dedicated practice can alchemize our relationship to even the most challenging circumstances, bringing stability, insight and meaning. The ancient wisdom of yoga empowers us to transmute poisons into medicines on the inner landscape.

Some adopt a yoga sadhana to connect more deeply with their highest spiritual truths. The fountainhead of yoga philosophy sees beyond rigid identities to the unbounded awareness in all beings. Yogic tools help strip away what divides us to reveal the sacred interconnection underlying everything. A contemplative practice exposes the peace, joy, and unconditional love resting quietly beneath our thoughts.

Of course, for many, it is an intuitive blend of all these motivations that magnetizes them to establish a consistent yoga ritual. Our original reasons for practice seem to unfold, expand, and transform over time as inner experience deepens. But reflecting on what calls you here and now allows intention to permeate your sadhana from the beginning.

Reconnect with Your Highest Aspirations

Take some time in meditation now to get quiet within and listen inwardly for the voice of inner wisdom guiding you toward practice. What longing of body, heart, or soul whispers to you beneath the surface layers of mundane habits? Let this work guide you toward clarity.

When ready, draw out your journal and write freely everything that surfaces internally in response. Don't censor or second-guess any thoughts or feelings flowing through – simply express raw and honestly to give shape to your deepest motivations. What are you seeking beneath it all in your soul's quietest chamber?

After fully downloading all that streams forth, read back over your exploratory writing. Highlight or circle 1-3 core intentions that feel most vibrant and magnetic to you now. Star any you sense will continue fuelling your will to practice despite future obstacles. These touchstone motivations will anchor you through the challenges ahead.

Choose one highlighted aspiration and artistically write it out on a blank sheet to frame somewhere visible near your practice space. This touchstone inscription imbues your practice altar with a sacred purpose, magnetizing the energy field to support inner flowering. Revisit this written intention occasionally when you need realignment or inspiration. Adjust artwork annually if core motivations shift.

Now contemplate your original framed intention and reflect honestly on the following:

How consistently are your daily choices aligned to this soulful aspiration?

Where might unconscious patterns undermine or limit this intention from blossoming more fully into reality?

What further changes would live from this intention require in your relationships, work, lifestyle, or use of time/energy?

What help or support might you need from loved ones to live more fully into this motivating purpose?

Who around you already models embodied living from a similar place of deep purpose?

A Mindful Path

When we commit to a new path, we must carefully examine where we stand now about our destination. Soulful yearning alone cannot transport us there. We must survey the terrain before us and become conscious of obstacles inhibiting forward movement. With compassionate self-inquiry, we can uncover inner blockages and external structures needing realignment. These revelations then illuminate where to focus our efforts along the journey ahead.

Awaken Your Unique Dharma

In the yoga tradition, aligning our actions to soul-given talents and passions is known as svadharma – expressing one's unique "way of righteous living." When personal choices and outer contributions spring from our essential nature, they flow smoothly as we ride life's currents in harmony. Friction and depletion often signal venues where we've strayed unconsciously from dharmic alignment.

Making course corrections then allows more easier self-actualization. As we grow into wholeness, we reclaim fragmented parts of self and step fully into an empowered purpose unique to us. Our personalized yoga practice can help shed obscuration around true dharma, so we know the right path inwardly.

What authentic strengths, values, and interests want full embodiment through you out in the world?

What brings you joy and feels effortless even amidst challenges when engaging your time/energy there?

Who seems constantly moved, touched, or positively impacted by your presence or participation?

What past pursuits left you feeling lit up, smoothly supported, and aligned to sacred flow?

Have loved ones or mentors reflected back soul strengths or talents evident to them but still unseen by you?

Consider the above reflections on personal empowerment and purposefulness. Then close your eyes and visualize your broader community as an interconnected web of light. See each person shining their unique gifts into the world like brilliant stars whose rays touch, inspire, and support others.

From this expansive bird's-eye view, pinpoint where your radiance wants to shine most vibrantly now for the benefit of all. What specific corner of the wider tapestry fits your soul-light offerings based on innate strengths and passions? The illumination you spread needn't fix everything; just uplift, nourish, and awaken around your small piece of the whole. When enough of us ignite thus, darkness recedes.

The Internal Spiritual Quest

Yoga means union – the fusion of individual consciousness with the Divine or Universal Spirit that lives through all beings. While each soul's evolutionary journey unfolds through unique choices and experiences across time, we're seeking deeper remembering of and realignment to our shared Source. All spiritual paths ultimately lead toward awakening from smaller egoic identity to rest knowingly in that infinite field of eternal peace and transcendent unity.

Regular spiritual practice serves to loosen and shed the veils of illusion keeping awareness shackled inside this tiny self-concept. Through contemplative tools like mantra, prayer, meditation, self-inquiry, or chanting, the doorway cracks open for Divine remembrance to dawn. In truth, we never depart from or reunite with boundless beingness – it is our timeless essence. But absorption in worldly matters occludes conscious knowing of this always accessible inner home.

A living inquiry thus awakens – "Who am I beyond roles, attributes, or experiences? What exists changelessly before senses, thoughts, or feelings?" As identity shifts from conditioned content to the unconditioned context holding all, inner freedom expands exponentially. We understand personal consciousness as a unique manifestation of an infinite, eternal Source from which everything arises. Realization blossoms that the same sacred essence living through this being also inhabits, animates, and connects all life.

The external practices of hatha yoga – its ritual movements, regulated breath, and stillness in meditative states – train awareness to remain centered steadfastly inside, withdrawing attention from the endless allurements and distractions of sensory existence. Through mastery of body and breath, the quicksilver mind rest in tranquility. This inward turn then ripens essential questions of higher purpose that spur genuine awakening from a smaller self to Sacred Self identification.

Clarify Your Commitment Now

With a clear intention set and preliminary self-inquiry complete, you stand on the threshold of a profound yogic journey toward wholeness. What must you now relinquish or release to step fully onto the path? Consider past patterns no longer serving next-level goals.

Where might self-defeating narratives still grip you? How will you reframe personal beliefs to align with your expanded vision? Do relationships require renegotiation around changing needs? How will you conserve energy for practice by simplifying demands upon time and attention? What hidden fears or resistances might future challenges expose for healing? A vigilant inner witness supports clarity around obstacles within and without. Make conscious deliberate efforts to identify and then release perceived barriers inhibiting your full commitment to practice.

Of course, no sadhana unfolds perfectly in a straight line from A to Z. Ups and downs are par for the course. What truly matters is continually clarifying direction and aligning choices to your True North. With firm, heartfelt intention seeded, surround this aspiration with a nurturing community to foster embodied flowering. Just one soulful friend committed magnifies inspiration, discipline, learning, and joy along the yogic path.

In closing this introductory journey of self-contemplation, crystallize your intentions for practice into concise seed phrases for remembrance:

May   this   sadhana   help   me

____

I   commit   now   to   prioritizing   yoga   practice   to

____

My   deepest   longing   through   this   sacred   work   is   to

____

Revisit and adjust such aspirational seed thoughts annually as your path unfolds. But for now, let them guide your steps forward firmly yet gently. Then, in stillness, feel through every cell in your body the quickening of destiny - a soulful prayer rising within toward living your highest truths. Here begins the journey without distance...

Sustaining any kind of yoga practice over a lifetime requires discipline and dedication. Fortunately, the tradition offers guidance for structuring a personal sadhana - a sequence of activities supporting mind-body harmony through ongoing self-inquiry. Building each day around simple yet profound rituals transforms transient inspiration into an enduring fountain of inner peace.

The first step in establishing a sadhana is identifying an appropriate practice space conducive to daily ritual. While occasional studio classes are invaluable, a home altar allows retreating into your private oasis amidst the chaos of modern life. Choose a quiet, comfortable spot and decorate the area with inspirational quotes, spiritual imagery, candles, plants, calming fragrances, or any other sensory cues signaling arrival into your inner sanctum. Allow this special environment always to remain a judgment-free zone filled with permission for self-care.

Just as important as the physical space is clarifying the optimal time of day for practice. Experiment to find windows of maximum alertness and minimum external responsibilities. Generally best on an empty stomach first thing in the morning; some may find advantages later in the day once work duties subside. Other priorities may force you to split time between morning and evening sessions. Lifelong consistency however depends on pragmatically integrating yoga time into mundane routines around family, work, and social connections rather than the other way around.

With consistent practice space and timing established, exploring the duration and type of activities filling this precious window prevents boredom and burnout. Most days include asana, pranayama, meditation, and study, though integrating other tools like chanting, ritual, or nature time revitalizes routine. Even just twenty minutes daily lifts baseline resilience, but consider building toward forty-five to ninety minutes long-term. Varying short and long sessions accommodate natural fluctuations in motivation and capacity day-to-day. End each practice with a dedication to merits toward universal betterment.

Checking ego and self-judgment at the door allows bowing deeply to inner wisdom. Come to your inner temple empty-handed, ready to listen and learn. Silence the tendency to constantly judge critically whether your performance meets arbitrary standards. Instead, bring an attitude of loving self-nurturance to even subtle inner disturbances revealed under yoga's microscope. Set the intention to study the patterns and tendencies of body and mind compassionately. This radical self-honesty and radical self-kindness catalyze rapid yet sustainable evolution.

Sustaining any kind of yoga practice over a lifetime requires discipline and dedication. Fortunately, the tradition offers guidance for structuring a personal sadhana - a sequence of activities supporting mind-body harmony through ongoing self-inquiry. Building each day around simple yet profound rituals transforms transient inspiration into an enduring fountain of inner peace.

The first step in establishing a sadhana is identifying an appropriate practice space conducive to daily ritual. While occasional studio classes are invaluable, a home altar allows retreating into your private oasis amidst the chaos of modern life. Choose a quiet, comfortable spot and decorate the area with inspirational quotes, spiritual imagery, candles, plants, calming fragrances, or any other sensory cues signaling arrival into your inner sanctum. Allow this special environment always to remain a judgment-free zone filled with permission for self-care.

Just as important as the physical space is clarifying the optimal time of day for practice. Experiment to find windows of maximum alertness and minimum external responsibilities. Generally best on an empty stomach first thing in the morning; some may find advantages later in the day once work duties subside. Other priorities may force you to split time between morning and evening sessions. Lifelong consistency however depends on pragmatically integrating yoga time into mundane routines around family, work, and social connections rather than the other way around.

With consistent practice space and timing established, exploring the duration and type of activities filling this precious window prevents boredom and burnout. Most days include asana, pranayama, meditation, and study, though integrating other tools like chanting, ritual, or nature time revitalizes routine. Even just twenty minutes daily lifts baseline resilience, but consider building toward forty-five to ninety minutes long-term. Varying short and long sessions accommodate natural fluctuations in motivation and capacity day-to-day. End each practice with a dedication to merits toward universal betterment.

Checking ego and self-judgment at the door allows bowing deeply to inner wisdom. Come to your inner temple empty-handed, ready to listen and learn. Silence the tendency to constantly judge critically whether your performance meets arbitrary standards. Instead, bring an attitude of loving self-nurturance to even subtle inner disturbances revealed under yoga's microscope. Set the intention to study the patterns and tendencies of body and mind compassionately. This radical self-honesty and radical self-kindness catalyze rapid yet sustainable evolution.

Setting micro-intentions focused on processes rather than outcomes maintains intrinsic motivation over time. Come to cushion or mat aspiring to simply reconnect with presence versus achieving advanced poses. When ego hijacks practice towards craving accomplishments, progress suffers. Let go of chasing elusive states like tranquility or bliss which arise spontaneously when we stop grasping. Instead, use the external form to deepen internal exploration in this moment without expectation.

Allow the practice to unfold organically from a matrix of wisdom, strength, flexibility, balance, and patience. Some days, energy flows smoothly while others feel uphill. Learn to modify, surrender, or get creative rather than bulldozing through resistance. By tuning into the body's signals with care and intelligence, over time practice traverses increasing challenges to build capacity and stability. Progress skyrockets when we drop unrealistic ideals of perfect practice.

Beyond quantified measures of growth, view setbacks encountered along the path as grists for awakening. Getting injured, losing a loved one, and career turmoil may all temporarily disrupt established routines. Expect occasional backsliding during life's inevitable crises. Staying gentle with yourself when overwhelmed or off-center prevents regrets and secondary suffering down the line. Even simple renewal rituals like restorative postures, walking meditations or pranayama reconnect intrinsic inspiration sure to resurrect full practice once the storm passes.

For lifelong adherence, periodically reevaluating the relevance and results of your sadhana protocol prevents complacency. Checking if chosen techniques still provide optimal benefits tailors the program to evolving needs. Certain limbs lose priority during stressful periods while other tools prove more essential than ever in times of turbulence. As progress unveils deeper layers of consciousness, additional practices integrate to navigate new terrain. Regular self-appraisal ensures you don't cling rigidly to paste formulas but remain responsive to your growth edge.

Staying open and humble makes space for unexpected upliftments. Routinization risks missing spontaneous moments of beauty, awe, or interconnection bubbling under the mundane. The same sunrise viewed for decades rewards appreciation anew today. Look for magic in simple sensations routinely overlooked. Creative insights dawn when we relax agendas. Allow yoga's non-linear alchemy to surprise you when least expected. What transformed yesterday's breakthrough into today's habit can elevate current plateaus again tomorrow. Each step along the path permeates consciousness with wider wisdom and freedom.

Prof. Mark Fanning

Chapter 11

The Psychology of Chakras: Subtle Energy Centers and Mental

Understanding the Chakra System

The chakras are an integral part of yoga's ancient wisdom, representing psychic centers of energy and consciousness in the subtle body. Far from mere metaphors or visualizations, a growing body of research suggests chakras may have real physiological correlates in the nervous and endocrine systems. While mainstream medicine is just starting to appreciate their significance, yogis have worked with these subtle energy vortexes for millennia as focal points for healing and transformation.

In this chapter, we will explore the fascinating psychology underlying each of the seven major chakras along the spine. Drawing from yoga philosophy and modern mind-body medicine, we will see how the chakra system forms an intuitive map of human development, encoded with profound insights about states of consciousness and keys for unlocking our deeper potentials. From the vibrant red of the root chakra to the radiant violet at the crown, traversing the spectrum between chakras gives us a holistic framework to understand and uplift the totality of our being - body, energy, mind, and spirit.

Prof. Mark Fanning

A rainbow ascending from earth to sky, the chakras personify our journey toward inner wholeness as we integrate progressively higher levels of awareness and purpose. While some portray enlightenment as a transcendence of this world, the chakra system affirms that we can advance profoundly in our realization while embracing every aspect of our humanity. Each energy center has vital resources for stabilizing and enriching our lives, from basic needs and emotions to perception, intuition, and bliss. By awakening the psychospiritual dimensions veiled within us, the chakras emphatically demonstrate we are far more than physical creatures subject to material limitations.

Filled with mythic power yet grounded in psychological accuracy, the chakras speak the language of archetypes that have resonated across cultures since ancient times. Human beings have long sensed we are beings of light and energy as much as flesh and bone, composed of mind and spirit as much as muscle and tissue. We feel deep within our subtle senses - intuition, inspiration, imagination - transcend yet permeate the mundane workings of neurons and sinews. The chakras give vivid form to this intuition, depicting our multidimensional constitution through universal symbols and imagery that awaken our higher identity. Subtle Energy Centers and Mental Wellbeing":

Balancing the Chakras for Wellbeing

A luminous spectrum reflecting our highest potential, the chakras symbolize the integration of matter and spirit, body and soul, in their ascending colors and properties. However, to unlock their gifts of consciousness and transformation, the energy centers must be balanced and aligned. Each chakra has associated patterns of physical, emotional, mental, and spiritual health - or disease - depending on whether it's functioning harmoniously or not within the system as a whole.

When the chakras are blocked or excessive, underactive or strained, we suffer disconnection from our deeper wisdom and vitality. Imbalances manifest as distorted attitudes and energetics pervading all dimensions of our being. We become disempowered and struggle with issues related to the chakra's archetypal domain, which may filter unconsciously into destructive habits or projections upon others. Healing comes from restoring flow and equilibrium to the affected energy center through developmental tasks, meditative focus, therapeutic modalities, and grace.

As psychospiritual conduits between body and soul, the chakras broadcast as well as receive, transmit as well as transform. They shape our inner state but also our presence and magnetism, which can uplift or disrupt those around us. Thus, balanced chakras benefit not only our mind-body integration but global energy fields we all share. Subtly yet profoundly, our private struggles or awakenings get amplified collectively by resonant waves. At this critical phase in humanity's journey, integrating and stabilizing our energy system serves planetary peace as much as inner peace.

The first chakra, Muladhara, holds energies of stability, embodiment, and feeling safe and grounded. When underactive, we may struggle with chronic anxiety about basic survival needs or our right to be here, take up space, and receive support. We might constantly feel threatened or undeserving without realizing that the root trauma or shame is fueling our stress. Healing the red chakra empowers us to embrace our bodily realm as a teacher, channel Earth's nourishing frequencies for self-love and security, establish healthy boundaries and transform fear into faith.

Prof. Mark Fanning

As the fountainhead of vitality and aliveness, the second chakra, Svadhisthana, carries adventurous, sensual, abundant qualities. Imbalances include emotional volatility, sexual issues, lack or excess of pleasure, confused or fused relationships, and crippled creativity from imprisoning social conditioning or past hurts. Getting energy flowing freely again in the orange chakra brings playfulness, embodiment, intimacy, and imagination to infuse everything we do with joy and meaning.

With its bright golden hue, the third chakra, Manipura, governs self-esteem, identity, and personal power in guiding our lives. When dysfunctional or deficient, we suffer from paralyzing self-doubt, confusion about our purpose, and lack of confidence and courage to convert insights into action. We might exert willpower through excessive control, domination, aggression, or narcissism as overcompensation. Stoking our inner fire harmoniously lets our core values and passion shine through to take authorship of our journey.

At the heart center, Anahata chakra integrates head and gut - intellect and instinct - with its caring, compassionate green energies. Out of balance, we cannot give or receive love skillfully, instead clinging or withdrawing emotionally while self-judging. We might rely too heavily on one-sided logic and lack empathy, and close-hearted due to grief. Awakening the heart's unconditional acceptance heals relationships by aligning us to our soul's perspective - seeing past surface fears and biases to goodness in all.

As a bridge upward from personal to transpersonal domains, the fifth chakra - Vishuddha - governs communication, authentic self-expression, and the power of our word. When blocked or disordered especially from criticism, limiting beliefs, or dismissing our truth to fit in, we cannot find our true voice. Instead, we may substitute meaningless chatter, deception, debilitating introversion, or refusal to address problems constructively. Getting the throat chakra flowing helps articulate our vision in direct yet compassionate ways that uplift others' spirits.

Beyond the balancing of each center, integrating the chakras' ascending spectrum is key for holistic well-being and consciousness evolving through its ranges - root to crown. As human development advances in stages, we shift identification and investment of energies from physical urges to emotional drives, mental concepts, intuitive wisdom, and mystical realization of pure formless awareness. Maturing into higher chakras' priorities and pleasures while keeping their lower supports, we stabilize high vibration.

Though shining at the head's apex, the sixth chakra - Ajna - represents the surrender of isolated ego rather than self-glorification or denial, as the opening and dissolving of personal finite identity into infinite spirit. Its gifts emerge from attuning to our indwelling spiritual intelligence behind thoughts. Hallmarks of disharmony are instead relying solely on logical analysis or external authority. Without integrating intuition, we lack deeper discernment and connection with our higher Self guiding us from within. Awakening the third eye, perception blooms beyond habitual filters to see all circumstances as lessons unfolding divine grace.

Finally, the crown chakra - Sahasrara - opens us to pure beingness, omnipresence, and the eternal now. We suffer when only identifying with time-bound sensations, thoughts, and circumstances, clinging to passing phenomena or fears about the future. Caught in the mental web of anxieties, judgments and incessant commentary, we feel desolate once whatever we were grasping as our sense of self falls away. But awakening to our boundless true nature liberates us to householder duties without losing transpersonal awareness - fully engaged in each experience yet not defined anywhere by limitations.

Prof. Mark Fanning

All phenomenal realms of vibration like waves on an ocean return to swimmers rather than swallow them.

By balancing knots in our energy system where consciousness gets stuck or scarce, the spectrum of chakras illuminates our path to embody ever-higher levels of vibration. Their awakening develops our soul's blueprint for actualization - knowing and showing divine being while excelling creatively through all centers. May we integrate their spectrum skillfully to stabilize peak experiences as our new normal.

While yoga asana physically opens and realigns the body, the system of chakras provides an inner roadmap for mental and emotional transformation. Chakras are vital energy centers linking the dense physical form to subtle layers of energy and consciousness flowing through the body. Each of the seven main chakras correlates to distinct aspects of our biology, psychology, and spiritual connections. When balanced, the chakra system fosters optimal well-being. When disturbed, these centers can trigger an array of mental health disturbances.

Understanding chakra psychology empowers you to identify the roots of emotional disturbances and employ targeted healing strategies. For example, excess stress often overstimulates the solar plexus chakra, depleting digestive fire and causing anxiety, irritation, and willpower issues. Practicing solar plexus-calming asanas like Bound Angle Pose helps retune this sphere. Alternatively, depression and grief commonly dam the heart chakra's vitality, creating feelings of disconnection and low self-worth. Opening poses like Camel and healing mantras progressively restore flow.

While chakras may seem esoteric, the latest research in mind-body medicine confirms neural pathways, hormonal glands, and organs strongly interact with emotional states and vice versa. For millennia, yogis mapped these mind-body connections through direct investigation of energy currents within the body. Consider chakras a codification of their empirical observations about psycho-spiritual stages of human development. Just as Saul McLeod's hierarchy of needs aligns with Maslow's chakra system, chakra maturation fosters evolutionary growth from survival needs into the actualization of human potential.

When aligned with the body's central energy channel or shushmana, balanced chakras calibrate nervous system function for peak performance. Distorted posture, toxic environments, emotional trauma, and negative self-talk can all throw this alignment off-kilter. Similarly, developmental delays or gaps in nurturing stages of chakra awakening manifest in adulthood as unresolved wounds or limiting beliefs about self-worth and potential. Using yoga to harmonize chakra flow smooths out these glitches.

The lower three chakras ground the foundations for safety, vitality, and self-confidence. The heart chakra bridges downward facing lower centers with upward-rising higher faculties. The flow between lower and higher chakras determines the mental bandwidth accessible for self-actualization. Free-flowing heart energy ensures full access to evolved states of consciousness. Next, the throat chakra externalizes our authentic inner voice and truth. The sixth chakra harnesses mental insight and intuition. Finally, when aligned, the crown chakra sparks awakening into cosmic unity consciousness.

Tuning into the subtle sensations and movements of energy within the body takes patience but amplifies the effects of physical asana. Simple practices like sensing each chakra during meditation or chanting bija mantras associated with specific centers enhance vitality flow. Performing vigorous or relaxing poses targeting areas where chakras reside also clears blocked channels. Any activity aligning your mind, breath, and body movements tunes the chakra instrument.

However, Asana is only half of holistically aligning this system. Cultivating the psychological qualities and elemental consciousness unique to each chakra ultimately balances their energy. For example, harboring chronic fears, playing small or excessively clinging for safety throws the first root chakra out of kilter. Getting grounded through community connection, financial stability or embodied confidence stabilizes foundation. Similarly, undisciplined work patterns scatter the third chakra's willpower while standing confidently in your values aligns with personal power.

Learning to trace emotions or limiting beliefs back to their subtle energy origins provides clues for holistic healing. If you commonly feel creatively blocked, follow that stifled voice down through the throat center. Rather than frustration, send compassion into places of tightness or contraction while engaging in opening practices. The patterns fueling stuck energies then organically unwind through sustained gentle effort. Meanwhile strengthening discernment melts away distorted perceptions clouding mental clarity at the third eye. Over time, fully living each chakra's highest expression manifests intuitive wisdom, unconditional love, and embodied liberation.

While modern medicine still debates the credibility of subtle energy theories, experienced yogis directly perceive the power of balanced vs. distorted chakras. Rather than rigid dogma, view the chakra framework as a practical model for optimizing bioenergetic patterns. Combined with other yoga tools, keeping your chakras clear and aligned accelerates awakening dormant dimensions of your full potential. Soon, you may even notice previously unseen connections between your psychological, emotional, and spiritual landscape, ushering in intuitive breakthroughs and conscious evolution.

Prof. Mark Fanning

Chapter 12

Diet and Lifestyle Upgrades for Mind-Body Health

The Link Between Diet and Mental Wellbeing

What we eat affects more than our physical health - our dietary choices also impact our moods, outlook, and mental well-being. An emerging field of nutrition psychiatry is making connections between nutritional neuroscience and psychology to understand better diet's role within a holistic, integrative approach to mental healthcare. As we explored earlier in our journey towards inner peace, wellness encompasses our entire mind-body system. Therefore, upgrading our diet and nutrition works hand-in-hand with lifestyle changes, mind-body practices like yoga, and the cultivation of positive mental habits.

Understanding Inflammation and the Gut-Brain Axis

Most people have heard the phrase "You are what you eat." More accurately, the microbes and nutrients you ingest impact far more than your waistline or risk for chronic disease. Research now shows the gut and brain intimately connect along the gut-brain axis, a bidirectional communication highway where messages sent from gut microbes can affect cognition, mood, and mental health. When we nourish our microbiome with a diverse, phytonutrient-rich, whole-food diet, these beneficial bugs produce neurotransmitters and compounds that reduce systemic inflammation. Unchecked inflammation drives the onset and progression of most chronic diseases, but also depression and anxiety disorders. Alternatively, a high sugar, processed, nutrient-poor diet feeds harmful microbes pumping out inflammatory messaging molecules. These inflammatory signals can travel anywhere, including up the vagus nerve pathway to the brain. Here, they promote neuronal damage driving mood disorders. Adopting an anti-inflammatory, whole-food diet provides the foundation for healthy digestion and robust immunity and can lift the clouds of mental malaise for clearer thinking and a sunnier disposition.

The Standard American Diet and Its Risks

Unfortunately, the average modern American diet deviates far from an ancestral, whole-food template in favor of hyper-palatable processed fare. This modern Western dietary pattern bursts with inflammatory advanced glycation end products formed when heat and chemicals alter the structural integrity of sugars, fats, and proteins. It also contains less phytonutrient-rich plant matter and relatively more saturated fats, refined grains, and sugars than traditional diets like the Mediterranean pattern. These now common industrialized foods flood the system with simple carbs, trans and damaged fats, and excess sodium promoting that problematic inflammation. They also alter communication along the gut-brain axis, change vascular reactivity in the brain, reduce the production of key neurotransmitters like serotonin related to mood regulation, and drive cravings for more junk food - creating a vicious cycle. Diet-related inflammation and these cascading effects now link eating this nutrient-poor, calorie-rich diet with increased risk for depression and other mental health disorders. So, while an occasional indulgence won't break the bank, making daily dietary choices that moderate these risks is wise.

A Mindful Path

Research Supports Plant-Based Eating for Brain Health

If the standard American diet provokes inflammation and threatens mental well-being, which diet proves more protective? Accumulating research suggests predominantly plant-based dietary patterns bolster brain and mental health through a variety of mechanisms. Plants provide high concentrations of anti-inflammatory, antioxidant phytonutrients; fiber to nourish a diversity of beneficial gut microbes; vitamins and minerals important for neurological function; and lean, clean protein sources. According to a 2021 systematic review and meta-analysis published in Translational Psychiatry by researchers from Loma Linda University, Oxford University, and other institutions across the globe, people consuming a more plant-centric diet had a lower rate of depression. Analyzing data from over 160,000 participants across 21 high-quality studies, researchers found nearly a one-third lower risk of depression for those adhering to a predominantly plant-based diet versus more omnivorous eaters. Plant-based diets are similarly associated with lower anxiety disorder incidence. Beyond this correlation with mental health conditions, controlled interventions also demonstrate eating more fruits, vegetables, whole grains, and beans while limiting meat and dairy also boosts emotional well-being, feelings of vitality, and daily functioning. Nourishing the body and microbiome with anti-inflammatory whole plant foods also feeds a happier, calmer mind. Time to eat more plants!

Benefits of a Plant-Based Diet for Mental Wellbeing

Transitioning to a more phytonutrient-rich, plant-centric plate better supports whole body health, including our mood and cognition. Here are some of the researched backed benefits of plant-based eating for mental wellness:

Prof. Mark Fanning

Improved Gut-Brain Communication: Filling your diet with a rainbow of produce, whole grains, beans, nuts, and seeds feeds the good bugs in the microbiome promoting intestinal integrity and facilitates healthier gut-brain signaling molecules up the vagus nerve to the brain.

Reduced Systemic Inflammation: Abundant antioxidants in plant foods stamp out free radicals and temper inflammatory processes associated with anxiety, depression, and cognitive decline.

Enhanced Neuroplasticity: Phytonutrients like the polyphenols in berries, leafy greens, coffee, and chocolate enhance neuronal connectivity in parts of the brain related to cognition, memory formation, and processing of emotions.

Optimized Neurotransmitters: Precursor molecules in plant foods boost the production of critical neurotransmitters like serotonin and dopamine linked to mood, motivation, and reward.

Altered Gene Expression: Compounds found especially in cruciferous vegetables like broccoli, cabbage, and kale favorably alter the expression of genes involved in promoting psychological resilience and an anti-inflammatory phenotype.

Cultivating Positivity & Purpose: Connecting to nature through gardening, farmers' markets, and eating seasonally localized foods can lift mood, inspire gratitude, and provide a sense of meaning.

Try going plant-based for just 2 weeks while also practicing your yoga and meditation, and see if these cumulative benefits resonate with your own experience! Even moderate shifts toward more veggie-centric plates with less meat pay mental dividends.

A Mindful Path

Adopting a Predominantly Plant-Based Dietary Pattern

Transitioning fully to a whole food, nutrient-dense vegetarian or vegan diet presents a tall order for most omnivores, as radically altering lifelong eating habits proves challenging. However, many prescribers in functional and integrative medicine now recognize a spectrum of plant-based eating, where your position relates to the percentage of daily calories coming from unprocessed plant versus animal products. Any gradual steps towards more plant-predominant plates help temper inflammation and boost mental health. On the strictest end, a vegan diet indicates 100% plants without any animal flesh or byproducts. Vegetarianism also excludes all flesh while potentially including eggs and dairy.

Further towards the middle, a flexitarian pattern emphasizes mainly plants while allowing a modest intake of poultry, fish, or meat. Mediterranean and Pegan diets fuse these flexitarian allowances for limited wild fish or fowl with strict exclusion of processed foods or sugars, emphasizing anti-inflammatory whole food plants, grains, beans, nuts, and seeds. Finally, those simply aspiring to eat entire foods focus on maximizing unprocessed anti-inflammatory plant staples, beneficial fats, and consciously sourced animal proteins within a well-balanced nutritional template. Each step towards more vegetables, fruits, tubers, legumes, nuts, and seeds incrementally boosts the anti-inflammatory, antioxidant, and phytonutrient compounds optimal for the body and mind.

While a 100% plant-based vegan diet rates anti-inflammatory and mentally stabilizing for many, it may not suit everyone's constitution or preferences. Most advocates just recommend eating MORE plants, not necessarily NO animal products if including them sustainably in moderation. Find your sustainable balance guided by how different ratios impact your energy, mood, cravings, and sense of well-being.

Incorporating More Fruits and Vegetables

Shifting from a conventional Western diet to a predominantly whole-food plant-based plate means doubling, tripling, or even quintupling your daily vegetable and fruit intake, which proves daunting for many. Having apple slices rather than chips, swapping a veggie smoothie for your morning milk and cereal, or trying zucchini noodles instead of wheat pasta represents easy substitutions to start where you are now with attainable additions you can stick with long-term. Before you know it, fruits and veggies become a major part of your meals and snacking! Simple dietary upgrades might include adding berries, bananas or avocado to your morning oatmeal or smoothie; quick pickled red onions, carrots or cucumbers for fiber and crunch on grain bowls or salads; roasting an extra tray of brussels sprouts, broccoli, squash or root vegetables to add into lunches and dinners throughout your week; tossing spinach or mixed greens into a wrap, sandwich, pasta dish or pizza weekly meal; sipping on low-sodium vegetable juices as an afternoon pick me up; blending canned pumpkin puree into marinara sauce, oatmeal or baking into muffins; taking a baggie of snap peas, mini peppers or carrots for at work or travel snacking; going for a vegetable first at dinner before modest lean protein and whole grains; swapping iceberg lettuce for spinach, kale or romaine on your burgers or tacos; and keeping diced tomatoes, beans, corn, and mixed vegetables on hand to quickly add into soups, stews, and chilis.

In tandem with doubling down on produce, transitioning to more whole grains provides essential fuel for the brain and beneficial fibers that feed our internal ecosystem. Refined grains like white rice, bread, and pasta as well as added sugars throw blood sugar levels off balance, promote inflammation and gut permeability, and ultimately negatively impact mood and cognition. Better to trade out white bread for whole grain seeded loaves; white pasta for brown rice, quinoa, or legume pasta; chips, crackers, pretzels, granola bars, and cereal for nuts, and seeds; roasted chickpeas or plant-based protein bars under 10 grams of added sugar; skip the white sandwich bread and go for a lettuce wrap or whole grain bun; choose corn tortillas instead of white flour shells; swap white rice for brown, wild, black or red hues; and limit added sugars through candies, sweetened beverages, and desserts.

Making half your daily grains coming from less processed whole food sources stabilizes blood sugar highs and lows. This prevents mood crashes from peaks and valleys in insulin and reduces the risk of insulin resistance driving inflammation. It also increases the intake of fiber, protein, and beneficial fats that bolster satiation. This equates to feeling full and fueled for longer versus rapid swings in energy and mood when simple carbs dominate your meals.

Prioritizing Legumes and Soy Foods

Beans made the food pyramid for good reason. All varieties of lentils, split peas, chickpeas and beans pack a substantial punch of plant-based protein, satiating fiber, key minerals like iron, zinc, magnesium, and potassium, and a spectrum of phytonutrients. Canned and dried options provide versatility and convenience as plant-based protein additions into a wide variety of dishes including chili, soups, and stews; hummus and bean dips paired with cut vegetables; quinoa, rice, and vegetable Buddha bowls; veggie burgers and meatless meatballs; burrito bowls; cold salads; and simmered in tomato sauce for a quick Bolognese. Having canned or cooked beans on hand enables easily incorporating this nutritional powerhouse into weekday meals.

Beans also contain unique bioactive compounds. Isoflavones in soy foods may support neurological health. Prebiotics in lentils, chickpeas, and beans feed beneficial gut microbes tied to reduced anxiety and depression through the production of anti-inflammatory short-chain fatty acids. Bean amylase inhibitors help stabilize blood glucose. Add affordable, shelf-stable beans to your weekly meal prep. Even quicker, grab canned lentils to toss into pasta dishes, soups, and salads for a no-fuss plant-based protein boost.

Seeking Out Smart Proteins

While transiting towards more plant-predominant plates, don't ditch all animal proteins if including them moderately supports your goals and constitution. Focus on shifting towards cleaner choices higher in inflammation-dampening omega-3 fats from pasture-raised animals, wild-caught seafood, and omega-3 fortified eggs. Don't sweat if sourcing or budgeting for better-quality proteins proves tricky. Stick with leaner conventional proteins in smaller portions as sides alongside antioxidant-rich veggies versus the main plate focus. Think 3-4 ounces per serving of poultry, seafood, or red meat a few times weekly rather than centering all your meals around these foods. gospel. Some smart animal protein choices aim for sustainability, ethical sourcing, and superior nutritional quality. These include grass-fed red meat over grain finished; wild-caught salmon in place of farmed; pasture-raised poultry and eggs from free-roaming hens; sustainably caught white fish populations not threatened by overfishing; grass-fed dairy over conventionally produced milk and cheese from cows fed corn and soy; and game meats like bison, elk, and venison managed carefully by wildlife conservation groups. Choosing meats, eggs, and dairy from small regional farms practicing regenerative agriculture supports local economies while providing superior community nutrition.

Targeting healthy fats across the dietary spectrum also helps temper inflammation and enhance absorption of fat-soluble phytonutrients. Focus on upsizing anti-inflammatory omega-3 rich additions such as olive oil; avocados; nuts like walnuts; seeds like chia, flax, and hemp; omega-3 eggs from pasture-raised hens; fatty fish like salmon and sardines; and coconut, ghee, or avocado based dressings. Emphasizing these plant and animal sources provides heart-healthy fats and essential fatty acids that balance the omega-6 inflammatory compounds accumulating from vegetable oils and conventionally raised meat.

Emphasize these beneficial fats while limiting pro-inflammatory omega-6-rich oils like corn, soybean, cottonseed, grapeseed, and rice bran oils, which are commonplace in processed and fried foods. Keep your total fat intake around 25-30% of your daily calories, and the scale should slide towards better mental health!

Nourishing the Mind and Soul Through the Gut

Remember Hippocrates proclaimed "All disease begins in the gut?" Two thousand six hundred years ago, Chinese Medicine also described the intestines as the "internal root of life." We now recognize the truth behind these ancient ideologies. Optimizing your internal ecosystem fundamentally connects to clearing the mental fog and lifting dark clouds hanging over your emotional outlook. Modern research illuminates the intimate gut-brain crosstalk where microbes and inflammation communicate via neural, endocrine, and immunological messengers. Fortunately, we can beneficially manipulate this conversation through intentional eating that feeds good gut bugs. Populate your plate predominantly with a diverse array of minimally processed anti-inflammatory whole food plants. Toss in modest lean proteins and beneficial fats most days. Then sprinkle in more yogurt, kimchi, kombucha, miso, sauerkraut and fermented foods boosting populations of anxiety and depression-reducing lactobacillus and bifidobacterium species. Limit added sugars, refined grains and factory farmed animal products prone to harbor antibiotic resistant bacteria and inflammatory advanced glycation end products formed under high heat processing. This whole food plant-centric dietary pattern with live fermented accents communicates positive signals up and down the gut-brain channel associated with enzymatic detoxification, downregulated stress response, balanced neurotransmitters, enhanced cognition and lifted mood.Implement these upgrades for 30 days as an experiment. Combine adding more yoga, meditation and breathing exercises over the same period. Assess for synergistic benefits that inspire lasting adherence to predominantly plant-based eating, mind-body movement and mindfulness practices skillfully merging modern science with yogic wisdom.

Establishing a Daily Meditation Practice

We've thoroughly covered how predominantly plant-based eating lays the nutritional cornerstone for balanced mood and mental wellness. Yet truly holistic mind-body health requires regularly pressing pause from busyness to reconnect through mindfulness practices like meditation. Luckily, just as one mighty oak grows from a tiny acorn, a few minutes of meditation daily over weeks and months cultivates consciousness and resilience. Through the simple act of sitting, observing the breath and recalibrating awareness from autopilot reactive mode to present moment receptivity, we nourish inner stillness. Consider meditation the ultimate nutrient for being rather than doing - quite the antidote for modern busy lifestyles!

A Mindful Path

The scientific literature clearly demonstrates meditation benefits brain structure, function and mental health regardless of spiritual belief. Meta-analyses link mindfulness meditation to enhancing executive functioning skills like focus, working memory and impulse control by thickening prefrontal cortex gray matter. EEG scans reveal different styles of meditation shift brain wave patterns in ways that enhance cognition, mood and stress resilience. Regular meditators also exhibit dampened inflammatory signaling, normalized blood pressure and changes in genetic expression related to circadian rhythms, metabolism and insulin regulation - all mechanisms supporting whole body and mind wellness. Whether participating in brief guided meditations or lengthier self-directed sits, spending this self-care time effectively nourishes inner peace.

Optimizing Setup for Success

Like establishing any new habit, setting the stage for success allows the seeds of meditation to take root then flourish into fruits of consciousness. This requires realism around your schedule, flexibility accommodating busy days, playfulness towards practice and compassionate self-acceptance when attention inevitably wavers. Arm yourself with realistic expectations around distractions and impatience before sinking into stillness. Establish a consistent practice that accommodates ebbs and flows. On tougher days sitting for even one intentional minute replenishes, while lengthier sessions may unfold organically on less hectic ones. View practice as a fun hobby versus strict chore. Let stimuli flutter in and out of awareness without frustration when concentration falters. Each sit still counts - there are no bad meditations! Remain ever grateful for the opportunity to simply BE present without needing to DO or change anything.

Identify Optimal Duration & Timing

Prof. Mark Fanning

While hour-long meditations certainly confer benefits, more practicable durations for daily life span 5-20 minutes. Those new to sitting often start around 5 minutes, gradually increasing until reaching whatever time frame prevents practice from feeling like a chore. Morning meditation links to lower stress and anxiety compared to end-of-day sessions. However, suitability depends on individual chronotype and lifestyle factors. Some love sunrise sits when minds remain tranquil post-sleep, while night owls might integrate meditations before bedtime when minds instinctively settle. Experiment to determine if mornings, mid-day breaks, or pre-slumber works best then consistently carve out this self-care space.

Construct Conducive Conditions

Before crossing your legs to sit in stillness, consciously craft conditions conducive to practice. Seek out a clean, quiet space permitting privacy from buzzing life demands encroaching focus. Turn off phone notifications and close computer screens, serving up endless distractions. Establish aesthetically pleasing ambiance through calming scents, soft lighting, serene music, or distracting white noise if needed to dampen external ruckus. Gather support tools like cushions, bolsters, blankets, and blocks easing any physical discomfort distracting attention inward. Sipping water nearby hydrates the body and brain while timed alarms softly signal practice completion. Prepping peaceful surroundings, even for brief stolen moments, informs the nervous system now signals sacred alone time versus continual doing.

Welcome Distractions with Equanimity

When attempting to focus attention inwardly as minds naturally wander outward, frustration frequently arises for beginners during meditation. Recognizing frustration itself simply represents another passing phenomenon noted, then released with non-judgment. Inevitable distractions like mental chatter, emotional surges, environmental stimuli, or physical discomfort all provide a grist for the meditative mill to reinforce present-moment awareness. Note distracting sensations, thoughts, and feelings as impartially as all other phenomena floating into consciousness. Avoid compounding disruption by layering self-criticism upon inability to focus. Instead, redirect to the meditative anchor using guidance like breath counting while adopting a gentler mindset through self-talk like "It's perfectly normal for attention to drift. Without judgment, simply return focus again and again to the breath". Progress transcends perfection!

Frame Practice Positively, Not as Punishment

Human motivation pivots profoundly based upon keywords held subconsciously. Framing meditation as "HAVE to," "punishing myself by" or "forcing myself to" elicits resistance undermining consistency. Alternatively, affirming meditation as an act of self-love, pausing from productivity or precious gifts we give ourselves invites engagement. Noticing subtle self-talk around practice exposes inner obstacles eroding enjoyment. Adjust mental messaging to uplifting intentions about why you want to meditate versus shoulds, oughts, and musts implying inner turmoil if skipping a sit. Lovingly begins again each day without criticisms around lapses. Inspired, patient practice outshines sporadic forced sessions over time.

Integrate Quick Practices Through Day

Lengthy, seated meditations certainly deepen awareness consistently. However, brief moments sprinkled throughout days, weeks and years also accumulate consciousness gains. Try quick, integrative meditations weaving stillness into daily tasks, like taking 1 minute to focus on the breath before checking notifications upon waking, which signals prioritizing presence over productivity first thing in the morning. You can also pause mid-commute as vehicles halt at red lights to relax tension through a few deep breaths before proceeding, set randomized alarms on your phone prompting 1-3 minute mini-meditations before moving to the next task, step outside for 30 seconds of fresh air with feet on the earth to connect to present surroundings spelled by sky, weather, sights, and sounds, or recall one positive interaction, accomplishment or personal strength at day's end before bed. Stitching mindful minutes throughout everyday life embeds the pause button necessary for responding consciously rather than compulsively reacting.

Mastering Meditation Mindset & Motivation

Beyond practical preparations optimizing daily sitting success, cultivating an adaptive meditative mindset maintains motivation long-term. What deeply held perspectives and beliefs either support or undermine your blossoming relationship with meditation? Radically accept the imperfect ability to tame the mind's wild wandering without self-judgment. Let go of fixating on tangible external signs deeming practice worthy. Instead, stand firm through phases of fruition and futility in recognition that mindfulness matters more than measurable metrics. Trust that sincerely setting intention plants seeds sprouting consciousness gains over time through daily tending - even when focused attention wavers. Water this budding inner sanctuary for the soul with compassion, consistency, and celebrations of tiny milestones toward stillness.soon bear fruits, flourishing into the fuller embodiment of inner peace with the mindful path walked step by step, breath upon breath through yoga's timeless teachings.

Overcoming Obstacles Along the Mindful Path

A Mindful Path

Like mastering any skill, advancing our meditation practice requires honesty, evaluating where we excel effortlessly versus feeling challenged. Without airing out dusty corners housing frustrations and limitations, cobwebs of stale mindsets and beliefs entangle our continuing education. Let's sweep clean mental clutter, undermining further progress! What common obstacles arise along the lifelong path of cultivating a mindful presence?

Procrastinating Practice

The paradox of meditation is that when we need it most, it is precisely when sitting sounds least appealing. Yet once anchored into the present moment, the clouds of overwhelm clear. When frantically trying to cram just "one more thing" into your overflowing plate before stealing a minute for meditation, pause first. Pressing on while mentally mazed rarely optimizes efficiency anyway. Instead begin by taking a few cleansing breaths, softening tense spots with conscious exhales then congratulate yourself for consciously choosing stillness in a dizzy world. Carving out mini mindful moments in the eye of daily life's hurricane winds us down while winding consciousness up long-term.

Trouble Taming Mental Chatter

One of the most frustrating yet ubiquitous meditation difficulties involves the endless stream of mental mutterings distracting attention from chosen anchors like the breath. Recognize rambling internal dialogues dominate waking hours for all humans, not some personal failing! Without beating yourself up, awareness continuously co-opted by mental movies simply signals overactive thinking brain circuits. Meditation slowly strengthens the prefrontal cortex "watching self" pathways, diffusing the barrage of thoughts.

Prof. Mark Fanning

When caught up in narrative memory loops, gently redirect focus to sensations of breathing. Say subvocal phrases like "thinking" or "distracted" to develop meta-awareness catching consciousness drifting. Accept that minds meander while commitment to redirect focus continually builds mental muscle returning again, again and again to chosen anchors!

Lacking Motivation Over Long Stretches

Beginners often leap zealously into establishing a meditation habit and then hit lulls where practice slides down priority lists. Remember motivation wavers naturally as inner work challenges the status quo. Stay sensitively attuned to leaks, slowly deflating your meditation bliss bubble. Coax consistency by consciously reconnecting to initial aspirations that sparked starting a practice. Recall precious memories of clarity, calm, or joy emerging from quietude. When sitting feels tedious, inject variety, trying alternate mindfulness techniques until one resonates. Seek inspiration from meditation MeetUp groups, podcasts, nature walks, or spiritual texts, kindling the inner flame when our willpower wick burns low. Yearning for depth again eventually flickers then slowly practice regains its pull. Trust cycles while continuing informal efforts through dry periods.

Struggling with Physical Discomfort

Establishing correct posture and aligning the spine while being supported by props aids meditative focus. However, tweaked knees from lotus pose to achy backs from slumping often plague beginners. Rather than gritting teeth to distraction in perfect picturesque postures, relax restrictions around fidgeting. Skillfully scan the body for tension almost constantly during sits by flexing fingers, circling ankles, and shrugging shoulders up and down. The release needs to perform meditation "right" by gently experimenting with simpler positions, easing any strains before abandoning practice in pain. If discomfort persists, explore options like kneeling pads, ergonomic stools, or lying down. Chronic issues may benefit from targeted stretching, mobility work, or professional bodywork before attempting lengthier sits. Choose what calms rather than conquers the physical frame so it supports rather than sabotages spiritual progress.

Stay inspired realize occasional obstacles encountered on the lifelong path and cultivate consciousness through meditation remain temporary. With wise, patient persistence embracing pleasant easy sits and those more painfully challenging, breakthroughs unfold. Relish small milestones like catching your internal mental dialogues through steps back from attachment to thinking self's stories. Savor those moments when cascading thoughts crystallize into a calm, abiding presence for just a few seconds - hints of the awakened state where liberation from suffering shines through. Trust each day's consistent efforts weave the thick mental muscle memory embodied over years that manages stressors with equanimity. Know that while a lifetime likely lies ahead to wholly master meditation, already your initial steps forward steep consciousness gains. For now in this precious breath simply celebrate small victories, directing attention gently back to the present. Then, without judgment begin again, again and again.

Designing a Personalized Mindfulness Program

While group classes and generic mindfulness apps prove useful in kickstarting meditation habits for many, custom-tailored home practices better cement long-term adherence. Carefully considering your unique life circumstances, challenges, motivations, and meaning reveals how best to sustain sitting through ongoing inner work. Co-create your mind-body wellness toolbox with evidence-based elements personalized for your needs. Then, interweave these mindful elements into existing lifestyle infrastructure through intentional habits planted, watered daily then blossoming on their rhythm. Here's how to organically grow a sustainable mindfulness flower in the garden of everyday life:

Start by identifying the priority intentions behind your budding meditation practice. What led you here - Reduce anxiety? Sharpen cognition for a career? Deepen spiritual connection? Now ponder how to continually reconnect preoccupations with those motivating purposes prompting practice versus typical autopilot living. Printing out inspirational quotes, affirmations or images resonates with visual learners. Auditory folks might record audio clips on phones, reinforcing why establishing mindfulness matters. Or keep a pocket journal jotting down post-session gains as well as obstacles overcome during the steep learning curve ahead.

The next layer is specific techniques suiting your leanings like mantra repetition for those seeking structure or open awareness techniques if drawn towards groundlessness. Balance passive observation alongside focused concentration skills working separate neural pathways. Then, determining the most accessible practice durations and seeing if pairing sits with rituals like pre-existing habits or schedule markers stakes the odds of following through. Three, two, or even one-minute respites summoning attention to the present sprinkled across days accumulate wins. The optimal frequency, style, and dosage depend on your aims and lifestyle. Customize accordingly then flexibly evolve practice as life shifts.

Further, personalize programming parameters with creativity towards realistic spaces serving up silence. Identify ideal spots like home shrines immersed in nature and quick spots sprinkled around daily paths for spontaneous sits. Think showering, treadmill walking, halting at stoplights, or during routine activity transitions already punctuating days. Myriad micro-mindful moments cultivate the meditation muscle memory required before longer sits feel alluring. Catalog options for formal seated sessions and mini-meditations are woven into the day's fabric when optimal settings remain scarce.

Finally infuse mindfulness into actions through informal techniques, blending inner stillness into outward tasks demanding attention like household chores, exercise and even interpersonal interactions. As Thich Nhat Han quotes "mindfulness means moments when we are there". What daily activities present arrive to anchor full awareness? Washing dishes, folding laundry, and meal prep all provide choiceless awareness training. Movement-promoting mind-body unions like yoga, dance, kayaking, and walking also teach tuning into subtle physical and emotional shifts from moment to moment. Even conversation and eye gazing offer routes to recognize projections we overlay upon present sense perceptions. Each hour holds hidden lessons in mindfulness. The wisdom unfolds through waking up while going about living instead of extracting exclusively to the mat.

Remember inspiration serves the short-term while discipline supports the long-term when designing personalized mindfulness programs integrated with daily living on and off the cushion. Diagrams depicting your web of extended mindfulness practice bring clarity around personalized pieces already established versus gaps needing to weave together increasing consistency, and cementing gains. Refer often to your unique blueprint when motivation dips, or frustration erupts. Having articulated intentions, techniques, durations, and locations supporting your continued progress shines light onto the next right action step when flailing in darkness. Rejoice realizing each effort unfolds self-knowledge, transforms consciousness, and liberates greater compassion towards all beings

sharing similar struggles. Our meditative blossoming ripples outwards helping collectively elevate global consciousness.
Cultivating Mindfulness in Everyday Life

Beyond setting aside exclusive time to train attention and awareness through seated meditation formally, we must ultimately infuse mindful presence into the mundane moments comprising existence if seeking abiding inner stillness. How fully can we immerse awareness into eating, moving, and even conversation versus just grinding through daily checklists preoccupied by planning towards the next task? As we learned practicing yoga postures, turning within revives vitality momentarily displaced by perpetual productivity. Regular redirection of attention inwardly to anchor consciously into the present also gradually percolates perspective rising above life drama narratives entangling the psyche into reactive mind loops. We awaken from destructive trances created by continually escaping now through anticipating future outcomes and ruminating about past events. Why trap consciousness churning misery over what no longer serves or cannot be controlled anyway? Instead, bring full awareness to experiences unfolding right here and now.

Daily life constantly serves up ripe invitations to practice receptive, mindful presence instead of resistant, ignorant trudging in unconscious autopilot mode. Rather than deprivation from external stimulation, cultivating mindfulness shines light onto knee-jerk-conditioned patterns driving dissatisfactory behaviors, damaging speech, and distorted thinking. Take that grating coworker constantly criticizing your efforts. Notice frustration burning your gut and how storylines project their nastiness as personal attacks entrench your inner angst. Yet by truly tuning into present-moment sensory input before overlaying perceptual filters, clarity crushes imaginary narratives. Try tightening facial muscles as harsh feedback fires then exhaling fully while relaxing temples perhaps exposed tension as their unease in role rather than antagonism towards your work. Prevention of habitual mental story spinning liberated by anchoring consciousness into current conditions via direct perception leaves little psychic space for toxic interpretations and drama-triggering reactions.

Choose Everyday Mindfulness Practices

Activities automatically activate a beginner's mindset fully immersed in just this moment and help habituate awareness-focused cognitive muscle memory-breaking tendencies towards trance absorption in critical concepts.

Each hour presents openings to either unconsciously lurch through another task anxious for activity completion or harness the space to activate mindfulness. Tuning into direct sensory experience, bodily movement rhythms, and subtle environmental shifts cultivates patience and prime perspective taking beyond egoic conditioning narratives. Be here now.

The Sacred Pause: Rest & Digest Lifestyle Rhythms

While momentary mindfulness interludes spark presence, regularly resting mind and nervous system from continual productivity modes restore sanity in frenetic modern environments. Humans evolved following natural cycles of stimulating hunts for sustenance followed by parasympathetically dominated digestive states promoting vital restorative bodily processes when the bounty is attained. Today's non-stop digital connections and pending responsibilities rarely permit such fluidity to flow between active doing and passive doing.

While yoga's mental and energetic practices provide a critical foundation, transforming your diet and lifestyle habits can accelerate progress along the path of mind-body health. The ancient yogis understood the intrinsic links between our outer world and inner landscape. What you ingest and how you live either enhances clarity or fuels disturbances. Upgrading certain key areas of your routine primes your system for stability.

Nutrition provides the raw ingredients for cellular function and vibrant energy. Eating to nourish rather than just feed the body regularly modulates its baseline biochemistry. Minimizing intake of heavily processed foods while maximizing fresh fruits, veggies, legumes, whole grains, and healthy fats optimizes digestion and assimilation of nutrients. Staying properly hydrated and minimizing toxins from artificial additives, sweeteners, and preservatives reduces metabolic stress. Herbs and spices like turmeric further enhance anti-inflammatory and antioxidant capacity. The yogic concept of mitahara teaches moderation in quantity consumed so your system focuses energy inward for healing rather than outward for digestion. Light, clean, sattvic foods balance the nervous system's excitatory and inhibitory networks.

Sleep is equally vital for resilient mind-body functioning. Yogic texts compare restorative slumber to the peaceful stillness of meditation. Getting adequate, regular, deep sleep allows nervous system repair and memory integration. The body secretes hormones overnight that facilitate growth and balanced moods. Skimping on sleep increases chronic inflammation plus emotional reactivity. Prioritizing a consistent sleep schedule pays exponential dividends in cognitive clarity and emotional regulation skills. The lifestyle framework of dinacharya guides optimizing daily cycles in harmony with nature's broader rhythms.

Beyond diet and sleep, establishing regular routines for movement, relaxation, and creativity further bolsters systemic resilience.

A Mindful Path

Whether going for walks, gardening, dancing, or practicing asana, frequent low-to-moderate physical activity stabilizes energy. Similarly, building in regular downtime to unwind tension via yoga nidra, listening to music, or time in nature prevents accumulated stress. Pursuing creative hobbies stimulates different neurochemical pathways than the daily grind. These lifestyle upgrades repattern your habitual psycho-physiological grooves toward greater somatic and psychological flexibility.

Upgrading relationships and building community provides critical social support for self-growth. Yoga philosophy recognizes healthy interpersonal dynamics as foundational to individual well-being. How we interact with those around us shapes emotional patterns - for better or worse. Reducing time with toxic people whenever possible minimizes a major source of stress. Deepening bonds with positive, sympathetic friends nourishes essential inner resources. Joining local wellness-oriented groups multiplies tools for thriving.

Cultivating simplicity and contentment in your financial and material lifestyle boosts lasting fulfillment. The concept of Santosha encourages appreciation for what we have rather than chasing external symbols of success fed by a culture of manufactured desires. Minimizing clutter in your living environment - physical, mental, and digital - provides space for clarity. Taming expenses to sustainable levels reduces the need to overwork to pay bills, freeing up energy for self-care and community.

Integrating mindfulness into daily routines grounds stable attention and Meta-awareness. Whether through short sitting practices, mindful eating/walking, or yoga, repeatedly interrupting unconscious perception patterns awakens presence. Pausing before reacting also short-circuits destructive impulse habits. Over time, this builds the muscle memory for responding skillfully rather than reflexively reacting. Regular reflection via journaling provides further opportunities to integrate lessons learned on the mat into wiser perspectives and choices off the mat.

While dietary and lifestyle factors alone cannot cure clinical mood disorders, optimizing these foundational pieces enhances the journey toward sustainable well-being. Strengthening outer supports allows inner transformation practices to penetrate deeply and irreversibly. With clearer biochemistry, space for renewal , and a supportive community, the light of expanded consciousness can steadily permeate layers of conditioned thoughts and limiting self-beliefs. Gradually, this recalibration process crystallizes an embodied sense of inherent wholeness accessible beneath all passing phenomena.

Chapter 13

Continuing Your Journey: Lifelong Learning On and Off the Mat

Yoga is a lifelong journey of growth and self-discovery. As you continue along the mindful path in this book, you will find there is always more to learn and explore - both on and off the yoga mat. Even after years of steady practice, infinite depths remain left to plumb within the ancient teachings of this venerable tradition.

In the modern world of instant gratification and quick fixes, looking at yoga as another fitness fad can be tempting. However, true yoga asks more of us than just showing up and perfecting the physical postures. To travel far along the yogic path requires commitment, patience, discipline, and an openness to continual self-improvement. Progress happens slowly, through small daily actions that gradually reshape your mind and nervous system. There will be plateaus where it feels like you have hit a wall in your development. Breakthroughs can also catch you by surprise if you stick with it. Building physical flexibility and mental resilience is an incremental process.

The key is establishing a steady, sustainable rhythm and not constantly comparing yourself to others. Avoid burnout by listening closely to the feedback from your body and moods. Be attentive but gentle with yourself as you navigate ups and downs in energy, flexibility, or mood. Over time, the simple ritual of rolling out your mat day after day provides an anchor of stability amidst life's fluctuations. Your yoga practice becomes the still point around which your growth unfolds organically.

Half the battle is just showing up with an open heart and mind. So be compassionate with yourself as progress waxes and wanes. Keep exploring within your window of challenge, but avoid pushing so hard you lose the inner spaciousness that yoga cultivates. What matters most is the spirit you bring to the practice. See each moment as a new opportunity to reconnect with presence. Your mat is simply the springboard into self-awareness - so also carry insights gained on the mat into all areas of your life off the mat.

As your yoga journey unfolds, be open to trying new styles, techniques, and teachers. Hatha, Vinyasa, Yin, Restorative - there are endless forms of yoga, each offering unique tools for self-inquiry. Testing different waters prevents you from stagnating and introduces fresh sources of inspiration to renew your devotion. Diversity also makes the practice more sustainable over a lifetime by working different parts of your body and mind. Though you may find certain lineages more resonant, staying flexible keeps you learning.

Exposing yourself to various teachers is equally valuable for gaining new perspectives. Every instructor offers their unique mirror reflecting back truths that you may overlook. Some may excel at alignment and the mechanics of posture. Others unpack the subtle energetics of prana and bandha. A few dive deep into yoga's spiritual heritage and philosophy. Most blend and balance different elements in their distinctive recipe. By sampling these different flavors, you gather more ingredients to nourish your sadhana as it marinates over the years.

Making yoga part of your daily ritual also connects you to a much larger local and global community. Practicing in a class allows you to inspire and be inspired by the dedication of your classmates. You realize we all struggle and have off days - permitting you to accept your ups and downs compassionately. Over time, familiar faces in classes become touchstones, providing meaningful human connections that sustain you along the winding road of life. Local studios also often host special events, intensives, forums, and training where you uncover new aspects of yoga's vast terrain at your own pace while deepening bonds with fellow practitioners.

This ever-expanding yoga sangha also extends far beyond any one studio or city. Today, more people practice worldwide than at any other period in history, yet we often only catch rare and fleeting glimpses into the personal journeys of these global companions. By reading books, blogs, newsletters, and listening to podcasts, you expand your perspective and feel connected to the worldwide renaissance and reinvention of this ancient tradition in contemporary times. Online courses also make teachings easily accessible from gifted teachers everywhere, continually illuminating new facets of this inexhaustible inner science.